MW00974169

$S^2O$
The Sexy Side of Holistic Health
Healing and Anti-Aging
LifeStyle Manual

My Personal Journey from
Cervical Cancer

## Dedication

I dedicate this book
to my mom
Gradey Carlathia Brown-Johnson
(March 29, 1941 – October 26, 2009)
I miss what we didn't share.
To my Dad
Chester Bernard Thomas
(May 17, 1926 – October 28, 1998)
Thank you for loving me enough to save me.
To my Daughter
Tatiana SeVon Jones
You are my greatest joy. The very air I breathe.
To my twin flame and mentor
I dedicate this book to all who are seeking.
Seeking what, you ask?
The answers to what you already know.
You have them. It's all inside of you.
To an all true and living God
Be the Glory!

# Acknowledgments

I want to thank my father Chester Bernard Thomas and my mother Grady Carlathia Brown-Johnson, my first teachers on this path.

Thank you to my daughter Tatiana S. Jones. I am always amazed and in awe by your sagacious spirit and your wide open heart. I love you so very, very much. Thank you for choosing me to be your mom this time around. ☺

Thank you to my siblings, Melvin Chatmon Jr., Vincent Jackson, Tony Jackson, and to my sister I never met, Connie Thomas. I love you.

I have a special acknowledgement for my biggest fan of a brother, Kevin Thomas (Ducky). Thank you for loving and supporting me, even when I didn't know how to give it back. You have always been there. I love you.

GiBi Brown, thank you for being there for me whenever I need you. You're so much more than a cousin. You're my big sister.

My constant and dear friend, Fadi Pattah. Time between us has no span. Thank you for everything

Diane Penchoff, you are such an angelic soul. Thank you for your love and friendship coaching me through my very first colonic experiences.

Dr. Stephen Brink, you paved the way for my exposure to *natural research and healing arts*. I appreciate you.

Dr. Sharon O.: Thank you for your guidance and encouragement. I now understand the gift.

Joya Summers: I would have never guessed our chance meeting would be the pinnacle in this book actually launching. Thank you so much Beautiful!

**To my mentors:**
Gabriela, you were the one to initially shake and wake my soul and kiss my spirit. Thank you for your stern words, your teaching, your touch, your unconditional love, your hugs and kisses.

My best girlfriend, Versandra Kennebrew. You inspire me. You never give up on me or let me give up on myself. I love you Sister.

My spiritual coach, Ma'at Seba. You made me think. Thank you for pulling the scales from my eyes to truly see ME.

My friend, Brian "B" McKissick – well I'll be darn. There you have it. Congratulations, but most of all, thank you for everything.

Jerry Johnson (JJ): I wish I could come up with a colorful parable like the many you share with me. Thank you for teaching me that it is ok use the *50$^{th}$Law*. As a matter of fact, it's damn near necessary.

Richard Vincent of ReEvolve Fitness: You launched my new paradigm in understanding fitness and personal development. Thank you for your guidance and love.

Saint Day Adeogba of YourDay ETC: Thank you for the experience. So much was learned. Would I go back and change anything? If it would not lead me back to here, no, I wouldn't.

Brooke Harbour of Transformational Health, LLC: I love you. Thank you for listening and sharing. You are an incredible woman, personal trainer and coach.

All of my YD Family: Tyrone McKinney (world's greatest Pilates coach) / Antonio Barnes (Sgt. Barnes – Super Model & Fitness Trainer) / Patrick Coleman (my island King & Fitness Trainer) / Trinity Williams (My Angel Girl & Fitness Trainer) / Aida Salmon (my celebrity skin care guru) / Sideeq Shabazz (you are love). Each of you made a chapter in my life transformational. I love you.

Ashley Riggs, Nick Sarnicola, Michael Craig and Ryan Blair of ViSalus Science: Thank you for your belief in me, your promotion of me and your love towards me. I know with certainty we will come together again, and it will be BIG!

Dr. Benjamin F. Baker: I sent out a prayer and the answer was you. Thank you for sharing. You have exposed me to so much. You inspire me to dream even bigger!

*Mother Father God and All that is Pure Love and Light, thank you for manifesting yourself through me as ageless health, abundant joy, financial prosperity and immortality. You are always conspiring for me to win!*

## DISCLAIMER

The advice contained in this material might not be suitable for everyone. The author designed the information to present her personal journey. The reader must carefully investigate all aspects of any health and wellness decision with their medical doctor before committing him or herself. The author obtained the information contained herein from sources she believes to be reliable and from her own personal experience, however she neither implies nor intends any guarantee this will work for the reader. The author is not in the business of giving medical advice, healing, or any other type of service. Should the reader need such advice, he or she must seek services from a competent professional. The author particularly disclaims any liability, loss or risk taken by individuals who directly or indirectly act on the information contained herein. The author is sharing her story here as her personal journey. The readers cannot hold her responsible for either the actions they take or the results of those actions.

# INTRODUCTION

Would you assume that experts use their information to your detriment? Well, they do. The so called "experts" bet on your ignorance and/or your indolence. It has often been said, if ever you want to hide something, put it in a book. However now, with the age of the information super highway, knowledge is immediately at our fingertips. Now the new adage is, if you want to hide something, make them work to find it. And even if we get the information, it may seem to be too much reading to even begin understanding the complexity of it all.

Instead, we choose to be in awe of the expertise of our doctors, lawyers, and government officials that we dare not challenge with inquiry.

Say you have been experiencing a headache for the past few days. You go to the doctor's office to check it out. The doctor rushes into your checkup room, ask a couple of basic questions and maybe feel your pulse and half-ass listen to your heart rate. Before you can fully explain your condition, he has his hand on the door knob ready to hurry to his next patient. Before he leaves though, your doctor will likely scribble a quick prescription for some pain pills.

That pill for the pain is only addressing the symptom, not the cause. ***Why*** are you having a headache? Your body is always talking to you, but when you numb it with unnatural substances (i.e. drugs), you can totally miss the whole conversation.

Here's another scenario. Say your skin is erupting in pimples, rashes and splotches. You schedule your appointment to see a medical dermatologist. She looks at your skin, asks a couple of basic questions and then prescribes a topical ointment to rid the rashes and stop the splotches. Again, the questions will likely not address your diet, lifestyle or water intake. There will probably be very little, if any conversation about *why* your skin is erupting. What is the root cause?

As an FYI, if you do have issues with your skin, it has been my personal experience and also my research has shown me that this is a manifestation of pressure from the liver not thoroughly flushing. Whenever I do a liver and bowel flush, it is amazing how my skin quickly clears up.

In an ideal situation, your doctor will ask you about your lifestyle, your diet, your water intake, your bowel movements and urination frequency. Ideally, your doctor would educate you about preventative methods to save your health. Instead of prescribing medication to cover the symptoms, your doctor would coach you into a better understanding of why your body is reacting the way it is. Once this understanding is gained, your doctor would then coach you through how to reverse the symptoms through cleansing, diet, and other lifestyle alterations.

Your body uses pain and discomfort to let you know, 'Hey, I got a problem here!' For me, whenever my head is bothering me, I immediately start working on getting my bowels to move. If my skin is breaking out, I will fast and do a liver flush. In just a matter of a day or two, my body is back in balance.

The best thing we can do for ourselves is stand in the responsibility of taking care of our health. Our health is our greatest asset and it is in our proactive participation in our personal care were we will find youth and vitality.

Too often I have seen opinionated, bull-headed men and women go out day after day, week after week drinking and eating any and every quick fix meal out of a box and spending very little time, if any to exercise. The only time water hits their mouth is when they brush their teeth.

I have watched many of my so-called "accomplished" friends drive their youth and vitality into the ground, all in the name of achieving career / financial success. Many of them are my age and even younger and they look much older. They are overweight to obese, graying, eating and drinking their way to high blood pressure and diabetes and joint pain, you name it. Mind you, most of my friends are not close to their 50th birthday! Some of them have not even reached 40! They are quick to spend their money on medications and the next fad or whatever that will keep them up with the Jones.

Then I have another collection of friends, a smaller group. They are also very accomplished world travelers and have been highlighted in various journals for their career accomplishments. The difference with this faction of friends is that we are very active. We weight train four to five times a week and we run five to ten miles a week, if not more. Most of us are vegetarians or vegans and we are vitamin / nutriceutical / supplement junkies. Most of us look ten to fifteen years younger than our actual years. We drink water like fish and we spend our money on therapies that will keep our bodies cleansed, our skin toned and tight, and our energy high. It's a really awesome group, focused on health. That in itself is sexy.

Now don't get me wrong. I don't want to come across as a purist. We party and enjoy life – unadulterated! We just do it in a way that is more supportive to our personal development and physical well-being. Occasionally, we may drink, eat and be merry, but you can best believe we are spending the following two days cleansing to get all of the toxicity out of our system.

To be frank, I lived most of my life as a part of the first crowd. I was ignorant about how to take care of my most prized possession – my health. I figured because I was young, vitality would always be on my side. I dogged my body close to death. I took the heredity of the habits I acquired from my childhood into my adult life. By the time I was 26 I was forty pounds overweight and dealing with some horrific digestion, elimination and female issues.

My friend shared with me a conversation he and his grandmother had before she passed away. She said, "*Baby, don't spend your money on anything that will hurt you.*" Wiser words could have not been spoken in that moment.

Hello and welcome to $S^2O$ - The Sexy Side of Holistic Health, Healing and Anti-aging Lifestyle Manual: My Journey from Cervical Cancer. This book was created to share with you my understanding of our body's ability to cease and reverse the aging process as well as cure and heal itself naturally.

It has been my experience that by reversing dis-ease, the body will also reverse and retard the aging process.

So many people are looking for the fountain of youth. You see it everywhere. I know for me, my attention was drawn to the glossy lifestyle magazines. Flipping through the pages and seeing the ads for tummy tucks, breast augmentation, liposuction and face lifts I noticed how everything looks sooo *sexy...smooth...youthful*. No wonder, even in these economic times, people are still willing to pay top dollar to sip (and snip) from the illusionary chalice of immortality.

When you really consider what goes on behind those slick ads, what could possibly be sexy about a steal blade slicing through your skin or a makeshift Hover vacuum piercing and gyrating in and out of your flesh, sucking out all the fat you put there? And let's not talk about the swelling, soreness, and high rate of infection. And one more thing to top it all off, they airbrush the models to perfection.

When I flip through the pages of some of my favorite holistic publications, the ads are soothing, peaceful and angelically serene. I could just float away on a billowy meditative cloud as I take in each visual of healthy wholesome goodness. However, I can't say the ads are necessarily...*sexy*. Functional and practical, but not initially captivating.

This got me to thinking. Many, if not all of the therapies and alternative healing advise

advertised in my favorite holistic publications
could definitely help so many people to
accomplish their desires of regaining and
maintaining their youth and vitality. Not only
could these therapies help, they could also
possibly save lives. I know many of them saved
my life.

I conducted my own one woman focus
group. I placed ads for tummy tuck and colon
hydrotherapy side by side. I also laid out ads for
surgical face lift and myofacial currant side by
side. I found that the holistic pages of serenity
could not hold a match to the professionally
tailored, model posed, filtered lighting, air
brushed advertisements of *"Get Your Snip Nip
and Tuck here"*.

It's unfortunate, because not only does colon
hydrotherapy support detoxing and cleansing, it
can also help with weight loss. I know for me, it
is amazing how my jeans are just hanging off of
me right after a colon hydrotherapy treatment. I
love getting a myofacial currant treatment. I can
immediately see the difference in my
cheekbones. They are higher and more defined.

I decided to do something to let people know
there are natural alternatives to health and
beauty. You can achieve that sexy, slick, svelte
body – naturally. *$S^2O$ – the Sexy Side of Holistic
Health, Healing and Anti-Aging Lifestyle
Manual: My Journey from Cervical Cancer* is

my "something" to let people know, you have a choice.

I am a strikingly attractive woman - tall, slim and appear much younger than my actual age. It's not just physical as much as it is that inside of me that shines through. This was not always the case. Amazingly, I look much younger today than I did 15 years ago!

I have appointed myself as the poster D.I.V.A (Divinely Intuitive and Very Aware) for the sexy side of anti-aging through holistic healing. Sound vain? Perhaps, but I believe that by the time you finish reading what I have to share you too will have another paradigm from which to recreate your life anew.

As a survivor of advanced cervical cancer, it is my hope that through my story you will recognize that you do have choices.

When it comes to health, healing and anti-aging the body does have the ability to cure and heal itself and reverse the aging process. As a matter of fact, aging starts from the inside out. Ill health is just a byproduct of aging. You want to reverse or cease the aging process? Work with your health and healing. Raise your immune system and consciousness. Suppressed emotions can manifest spiritually, mentally, and eventually physically. Your emotions are part of your consciousness and your consciousness creates.

Every part of the dynamic machine you live in is inner connected; mentally, emotionally, spiritually and physically.

My intention is to share my understanding of this inner weave of connectivity to empower you to study further on your own and implement some of the teachings into your personal lifestyle.

It is very important to understand, what you put in your body can have a long lasting effect. What you listen to (music). What you watch (television). What you feel (emotion) can and will shape and mold your life. How your life unfolds is all in your hands.

I cannot express the importance of your thoughts. Your thoughts will lead to your feelings. Your feelings will lead to your actions and your actions will lead to your outcome. What you think and feel has an even greater effect on your vitality, health, well-being and wealth than what you perform in action.

In this book, I share my current understanding from personal experience about nutritional supplements and holistic therapies that you may find very beneficial. These therapies and supplements have become the staple of my lifestyle and support the maintenance of my youth, vitality and my sex appeal.

Getting older and aging is not the same thing.
- Getting older relates to the passage of time.
- Aging relates to the breakdown of tissues in the body.
- The outward signs of aging include wrinkles, sagging, and gray hair.
- Getting older by itself does not cause aging.

This manual has been indexed in three parts.

1. The first index is my personal life sprinkled with some antidotal stories that helped me to observe myself through others. I candidly share my journey to and through my diagnosis of advanced cervical cancer. I have also shared some simple yet powerful exercises that have helped me along my journey.

2. The second index is the therapies that I utilized during my transition of healing, with my interpretation of what the therapies are and how they helped me. I have also noted the supplements I used then and what I use today as a part of my holistic anti-aging lifestyle maintenance program.

3. And the third index is a resource guide listing of websites to gain additional information in your search.

PLEASE NOTE: Listed in this lifestyle manual are my personal opinions based on my experiences and are not to be misconstrued as a form of treatment for any dis-eases. The resource guide is drawn from my personal experience and extensive research of various nutritionals, supplements and therapies.

Before you begin any wellness regimen, consult with your physician or wellness professional.

Thank you for this opportunity to share my story. I bid you...LIFE! Live – Without Reservation or Apology.

# TABLE OF CONTENTS

## INDEX I

# INDEX II

# INDEX III

# INDEX I
# Chapter One

## PROGRAMMED BELIEFS

I have spent too many of my adult years in needless suffering because of my programmed beliefs in things like:

*"Because my mother and father had high blood pressure / cancer / diabetes I will too."*
This is total kaa-kaa!

*"I have to take medication for my depression."*
Sure, and become num in the process to any kind of emotional sensation.

*"If my body begins to show signs of aging I had better prepare for an ongoing maintenance of surgeries to stay looking young."*
Oh sure, and end up looking like the Cat Lady scaring small children and forest animals. Hey why not just turn my face into a human needle cushion for botox injections? Yeah! NOT!!

*"I could never forgive, let along forget what my so called best friend did to me. I will take what she/he did to me to my grave!"*
That which you speak so shall it be! Hold on to all of that old mess if you want to. She/He has totally moved on and likely not even thought twice about the whole event anyway. Or even better yet, has no idea that what they said or did

had such an impact on you. Here it is 476 years later and you are still lamenting over that mess???

*"In order to be successful, I will have to work very hard."*
Not even necessary! As a matter of fact, how many people do you know that have nearly worked themselves into their own grave? It does not matter how much money you make, if you do not have your health and inner joy, the measure of success can be futile.

*"I can't give up my chit'lins, pork skins, and T-bone steaks. And you're tellin' me to put down my soda pop too? Dang, what am I suppose to eat and drank? (This is not a typo, yes drank)*
Did you know that the body typically has a hard time digesting animal flesh? Red meat actually has to rot in your gut before it can break down to flush out…providing it flushes out at all! And soda? The carbonation is actually pulling the calcium from your bones, which is probably part of the reason why you are experiencing the joint pain and bone deterioration. Oh and if you're drinking diet soda... it's making you fatter.

This is not even the tip of the iceberg of some of my old beliefs that I had to shatter. I could go on and on about how many disappointments and failures I have encountered because of what he/she should have, would have, and could have done for me. Nobody knows the troubles I've seen – Nobody knows my sorrows.

*[Enter here symphony violins, dramatic effect and Kleenex tissue box.]*

These thoughts are limiting. **We are not at all limited** and I have proof… tons of proof, as I am living it!!

I have a few questions for you:

- Is your health affecting your happiness and joy in life?
- Are you constantly replaying painful life scenarios repeatedly in your mind from long past?
- Are you spinning in a sense of despair and deep depression?
- Are you living hand to mouth without recourse for economic sovereignty?

This was my life. **I was living in past paradigms that were long from serving me**. In my strong will to hold on to "being right", my health was held by the glorified prison of my self righteous false ego fore, **I** was just…**I** was right! Of course, my joy and financial freedom also followed suit of my health.

**I** was the one done wrong by… you name it—my mother, my father, my siblings, my 3$^{rd}$ grade teacher, the bum that cut in front of me on the highway, the pigeon that crapped on the shoulder of my new leather jacket. Shall I go on?

I was holding onto so much unnecessary emotional garbage. Just the thought of any one of my little emotional upsets, and I could feel my blood pressure rising and my face heating up with anger.

What's crazy is that I lived my life like this consistently for so long my body was in a perpetual state of tension. Brewing over my emotions, my physical health was more than questionable and I was dealing with bouts of depression that at times bordered suicidal tendencies. I had no idea of how to handle my emotions other than to bury and just keep them suppressed. However I soon learned from a fascinating book I picked up a few years ago titled, *Feelings Buried Alive Never Die* by Karol K. Truman, that I was doing more harm to myself (and others) than good. Not only do those pesky little firebombs of ill sentiments eventually rear their ugly little heads in the heat of any given situation where you really need to

*In times of change the learners shall inherit the earth while the learned will find themselves beautifully equipped to deal with a world which doesn't exist.*

keep your cool, the energy from them will create tension in your body as well creating the perfect environment for dis-ease to fester. I go a bit more into this later in the book.

# Chapter Two

## DIAGNOSIS CANCER / PROGNOSIS 3-6 MONTHS

I was diagnosed with advanced cervical cancer and given a prognosis of 3-6 months. This was about eight years ago. My options… exceptionally few with no guarantee

> *It wasn't until I was standing in the face of death that I truly decided to LIVE!*

to take me beyond the short timing of what was to be my final fate.

It's amazing how I began to look at life so differently. It's almost comical to think that at one time or another I considered terminating my life. When I think about this I just have to shake my head and laugh at myself.

It's sorta like how a child would react to a toy that has been broken. Me breaking my toy is one thing, but someone / something else threatening to break my toy, well now you've got a fight on your hands. I guess it's just human nature.

All I knew is that I wanted to live. This event took me totally out of my pity party and set me straight. This event and strong words from my mentors.

It was time to make some decisions about my life and what I decided… I wanted to LIVE!

In the midst of this confusing time, my mind was clear enough to know that I did not want to relinquish myself to conventional modalities. Prior to all of this drama, I had picked up a book or two here and there and had acquired just enough information to understand that the body has the ability to cure and heal itself. I just had to find out how. In greater part, I came to this conclusion because of my father and a message I received during a meditation.

### About My Father

You see, in 1998, my father passed away from complications that manifested into prostate cancer. I bore witness to a handsome, active man of 6'2" stature, wither away by the ravenousness of bonded emotions, poor diet, radiation and drug therapy.

### My Message in Meditation

I prayed. In my conversation with God, I asked for guidance and clarity in understanding. I meditated. I listened for a response to my quest. Just as clear as a conversation I would have with you face to face, I heard a voice. "What are your needs?" I thought, "My needs? I need my health and money to pay for my health?" Calmly the voice said to me, "Write down your needs." To not lose the moment, I ran to get a pad and pen and sat back down patiently waiting for further instruction. Again, "Write down your needs." So, I wrote down:

I need my health.

I need money to pay for my health.

I need…

**I** stopped writing. It was as though something gently came over me and took lead. What was written on the pad…

$$N$$
$$E$$
$$E$$
$$D$$
$$S$$

On letter underneath the other. I looked at the writing – and then the "lead" continued:

**N**utritional

**E**ducational

**E**motional

**D**etox

**S**piritual

Just as gently as "it" came, "it" gently left, so I suspected. I looked at my pad with curiosity and surprise. It made sense.

At this time, I was physically fatigued, spiritually drained, and financially busted. I pushed on to take care of my teenage daughter, and even this was a challenge as our relationship was strained at best. My emotions literally riddled my body with stress.

I just knew something had to break loose. From where I was, there was only one way to go, and that was up.

My casual curiosity fired into a full time quest. I began to research and read. You name it I have probably read it -- alternative health, organic food preparation, energy balancing, motivation, inspiration, morning dedications. If you ever want to know how to prepare a blessed head of healthy month old cabbage cider to clear your chakras – give me a ring. I got cha covered!

I attended seminars and classes getting bits and pieces of what I needed from every one of the great masters of physical healing, self empowerment and motivation.

All this frickin' enlightenment cost me a mint! Some of this information has become the staple of my success, other parts that did not serve me at the time, I tossed only to pick it up and implement it into my life at a later time that was more appropriate.

I inundated myself with information, but none of it provided the Holy Grail to the aesthetically polished immortals I saw airbrushed in the glamour magazines with their perky breasts and glowing skin. Nor did I gain the Rob Report lifestyle of Polo plaid golf skorts with the matching pink button down cardigan.

At this point, all I wanted was my health - my health and something – anything that resembled happiness.

I didn't want much. Not at all! Heck, I'm a good person. Why couldn't I just have a little peace!!

Here I was, damn near 40 years old and very little to show for it. My energy was low, and my life force was fading quickly.

To keep my mind off of everything that was going on with me, I was working long hours at a job that I didn't like – Correction. I HATED IT!! And I struggled financially. I was anything but healthy, joyful and prosperous, like the gurus told me I could be. I had just about given up on life.

### My First Spiritual Mentor

I met and befriended this absolutely enchanting German Hungarian Gypsy. Her name is Gabriela and she is beautiful! Gabriela has dark raven hair and fire brown eyes. Her smile and her personality pulled me right in. She has the type of energy that is infectious and you want to be around her.

Gabriela pulled me over to the side one day after listening to me moan, groan and bitch about what I didn't have because of so n' so and such n' such. She got totally in my face and with her thick broken English, German accent, she said, *"You need to make up your mind. Either make change or play victim sheep and be herd through your own pitiful slaughter! Apply what you know, or you know nothing!"*

Her words were stern, but they had to be in order to wake me up. The final ingredient of the formula awakened the

*When the student is ready, the teacher(s) will appear.*

beginning of transformation in my life resulting in the gain of my health (physically, emotionally, and spiritually), and charging me with boundless joy. I took responsibility and applied my knowledge.

Another thing that Gabriela shared – she told me that if I would allow my heart to be open and pay attention, the Universe (God) will speak to me. You know what? She was right!

**315**
315 is a very significant number to me. My birthday is March 15th. I began to notice that everywhere I looked, I saw 315 – on license plates, the clock on the wall, the address on a building. God was talking to me and giving me confirmation through our own little secret code. 315.

As my awareness strengthened, there was a clarity that surfaced and allowed me to bring to fruition stages of health, joy and prosperity that continues to grow.

Along this journey I found the fountain of youth. I look and feel better now in my 40s than what I ever did in my late teens and early 20s. I'm looking forward to my 50s!

Many of the therapies I employed, the diet I adhered to and the supplements I took during my healing rehabilitation, I still use in my daily regimen.

My adopted lifestyle keeps my skin youthful and my body toned and tight. My energy is up, my mind is sharp and focused and my "nature"...playful. I run circles around young girls more than half my age.

Because my energy is high, I attract people and situations to me that are of the same caliber. How my life was eight years ago and beyond is like a shadow compared to how my life has unfolded since then.

Youth, vitality, sexuality, weight loss, complete health, joy and even prosperity...these are not things you find in a doctor's office under the blade of a knife. These are not experiences you will dig from underneath the cotton puff of pill bottle. Neither will you find it by giving away your power to the doctors, telling them to fix what you have used YOUR power to break down.

You have more control over your health and well-being than you would ever know, or maybe want to accept responsibility for.

# Chapter Three

### TRANSFORMATION / TRUTH / LOVE

My health turned around 180°. When I went back to the doctor 10 months later after my initial diagnosis and prognosis, the grapefruit size infection they originally found on my cervix had reduced to the size of a lima bean. The six fibroid cysts – all gone and this is without surgery, radiation, chemo, or drugs.

For the first time in my life, I was clear of my purpose and focused on my direction. Life transformed into something absolutely magical.

**All this, from just making a decision- a decision to <u>take responsibility</u> for my health, my healing
MY LIFE!**

Not everyone is prepared to accept the TRUTH. The truth can sometimes hurt. If you are *What is TRUTH?* not ready for the truth, you will undoubtedly find yourself closing this book and setting it aside. Then too, each of our versions of truth differ, one from another.

What may be truth for me may not be truth for you.

What may be truth for you now may not be truth for you five years from now. It may not even be truth for you five days from now – fives hours, or even five minutes!

One thing for certain though, life keeps going and depending on where you are in your life, what may have been fitting for you back in the day, may not be applicable now.

Case in point: As I was entering into my adult years, I was extremely angry with my mother and father. I felt that they should have, could have, if only they would have, I would be X, Y, and Z.

I was not in the place to take responsibility for myself. It was easier to blame everyone else for my unhappiness and misfortune.

For the longest I blamed my parents for my misery and how my life had turned out. Then I came into a new understanding. Mom and Daddy did the best they could do with the life tools they had to work with. I had to take responsibility for my existence and make a determination as to how I wanted my life to play out.

> *You are not responsible for changing, fixing or transforming anyone but YOURSELF!*

Once I took the reins of my life I began applying my knowledge. Instead of adding things outside to me to feel better, I dwelled on my inner being. Besides, buying stuff (i.e.

clothes, jewelry, cars, etc..), only gave me a temporary joy and long term debt.

This shift in me allowed an environment of understanding and forgiveness of MYSELF and others. With my new understanding it was easier to let go of the blame and judgment that I was directing toward everyone else.

This evolution has brought me through and continues to groom me for an unconditional acceptance of all people, especially myself.

As I chose to accept each individual (including myself) where they are and the way they are, it is in each and every moment I share an unconditional understanding and like magic everything and everyone outside of me transforms too.

### Aging / Dis-ease: It's a Decision
I came across an awesome story by George G. Ritchie, *Return from Tomorrow*. I took an excerpt from his book that I want to share this with you.

*When the war in Europe ended in May 1945, the 123$^{rd}$ Evac entered Germany with the occupying troops. I was part of a group assigned to a concentration camp near Wuppertal, charged with getting medical help to the newly liberated prisoners, many of them Jews from Holland, France and Eastern Europe. This was the most shattering* *experience I had yet had; I have been exposed many times by then to sudden death and injury, but to see the effect of slow starvation, to walk through those barracks where thousands of men had died a little bit at a time over a period of years, was a new kind of horror. For many it was an irreversible process: we lost scores each day in spite of all the medicine and food we could rush to them.*

*And that's how I came to know Wild Bill Cody. That wasn't his real name. His real name was several unpronounceable syllables in Polish, but he had a long drooping handlebar mustache like pictures of the old western heroes, so the American solders called him Wild Bill. He was one of the inmates of the concentration camp, but obviously he hadn't been there long; his posture was erect, his eyes bright, his energy indefatigable. Since he was fluent in English, German, French, Russian and Polish, he became a kind of unofficial camp translator.*

*We came to him with all sorts of problems; the paper work alone was staggering in attempting to relocate people whose families, even whole hometowns, might have disappeared. But though Wild Bill worked fifteen and sixteen hours a day, he showed no signs of weariness. While the rest of us were dropping with fatigue, he seemed to gain strength. 'We have time for this old fellow', he'd say. 'He's been waiting to see us all day.' His compassion for his fellow-prisoners glowed on his face, and it was to his glow that I came when my own spirits were low.*

*So I was astonished to learn when Wild Bill's own papers came before us one day that he had been in Wuppertal since 1939! For six years he had lived on the same starvation diet, slept in the same airless and dis-ease ridden barracks as everyone else, but without the least physical or mental deterioration.*

*Perhaps even more amazing, every group in the camp looked on him as a friend. He was the one to whom quarrels between inmates were brought for arbitration. Only after I'd been at Wuppertal a number of weeks did I realize what a rarity this was in a compound where the different nationalities of prisoners hated each other almost as much as they did the Germans.*

*As for Germans, feelings against them ran so high that in some of the camps liberated earlier, former prisoners had seized guns, run into the nearest village and simply shot the first Germans they saw. Part of our instructions was to prevent this kind of thing and again, Wild Bill was our greatest asset, reasoning with different groups, counseling forgiveness.*

*'It's not easy for some of them to forgive,' I commented to him one day as we sat over mugs of tea in the processing center. 'So many of them have lost members of their families.'*

*Wild Bill leaned back in the upright chair, sipped at his drink slowly and uttered the first words I had heard him speak about himself, 'My wife, our two daughters, and our three little boys. When the Germans reached our street they lined everyone against a wall and opened up with machine guns. I begged to be allowed to die with my family, but because I spoke German they put me in a work group.' He paused, perhaps seeing again his wife and five children. 'I had to decide right then,' he continued, 'whether to let myself hate the soldiers who had done this. It was an easy decision, really. I was a lawyer. In my practice I had seen too often what hate could do to people's minds and bodies. Hate had just killed the six people who mattered most to me in the world. I decided then that I would spend the rest of my life – whether it was a few days or many years – loving every person I came in contact with.'*

This story moved me. Wild Bill lived the same starvation diet, slept in the same airless and disease ridden barracks as everyone else, BUT –

without the least physical or mental deterioration.

Obviously Wild Bill acquired tools – spiritual and emotional tools to help him overstand the real truth of the matter. There is no higher vibration than love and no higher calling than the calling to forgive, serve and heal.

**What's in Your Tool Box**

Standing on the foundation of unconditional love and forgiveness requires some serious emotional and spiritual tools. Let's say you need to build a house, but if the only tool you have in your toolbox is a hammer, you will find the process of building your home a bit challenging, at best. Certainly, you need the hammer, but do you need the hammer to cut the wood or lay the bricks? Would you use the hammer to install the glass windows?

My grandparents (both my Mom's folks and Daddy's) did the best they could do with raising my parents. They used what tools they had in their (mental, emotional, spiritual) toolboxes to raise their children. In turn, my parents did the best they could do with what they had. It was up to me to expand my own tool box.

In order for me to fully live my life, I had to let go. Let go of the past hurt, pain, and fears. Had I continued to spin in that energy of anger and bitterness, I would surely be dead - eventually physically and definitely spiritually and emotionally. My personal experience has questioned whether ongoing emotional pain could be worse than death itself. I would say yes, because at least in death there is greater possibility for rest.

Keep in mind - **continue to do what you have always done, you will get what you have always gotten.**

Are you using the right tools to build your temple of understanding, patience and forgiveness? What is your truth right now? What are you holding onto that isn't serving you?

As you take inventory of your life, be truthful with yourself. If you were to continue on the path you are currently on are you satisfied with the fact that things will remain in this same paradigm?

You are the architect of your life. How you build from here is up to you. Gather your tools wisely.

*Negative feelings, thoughts and attitudes will rob your well-being. Positive feelings, thoughts and attitudes feed, nourish and sustain your health.*

# Chapter Four

**EXERCISE I**

Heartbreak is not the easiest thing to get over. Heartbreak does not necessarily happen from a lover or a spouse. A heartbreak can involve anyone you put your trust in.

Sit back and think for a while. What are your top three heartbreaks that keep replaying in your mind?

1. Who broke your heart? _____
What happened: _____

_____

_____

_____

_____


2. Who broke your heart? _____
What happened: _____

_____

_____

_____

_____


3. Who broke your heart? _____
What happened: _____

_____

_____

_____

_____

Everything is one thing – ENERGY. Emotion is energy. E + Motion = Energy in Motion. Sickness and dis-ease always begin as something you cannot see, E-motion: Energy in motion. Over a period of time, when you are experiencing the same degenerating reaction over and over again (anger / anxiety / worry), it develops into something that you feel (i.e. headache / backache / stomach problems). As time continues on and changes are not made to convert the e-motion, the energy compounds, creating ulcers, chest pain, and even more serious physical manifestations.

You have no doubt experienced your heart pounding, a knot in your stomach, extreme nervousness, insomnia, impatience, anger and anxiety. Likely, you have just come to accept these conditions as a part of getting through the day and have just labeled the physical experiences as STRESS.

The effects of your stress are much more insidious than you realize. According to Dr. Paul J. Rosch, former president of the non-profit American Institute of Stress in Yonkers, NY, the stress in the United States is taking a terrible toll on the nation's health and economy. Stress contributes heavily to heart dis-ease, respiratory distress, cancer, lupus and numerous other life-threatening dis-eases. It is one of the primary reasons for the astronomic health-care costs in the United States. And yet, stress is very difficult to define because it varies with each individual.

Stress and how you handle it can always be traced back to the early conditioning / training that contributed to your feelings and beliefs (i.e. childhood). While striving to overcome a particular stress, you will want to be mindful of what is happening inside your body. Ask yourself, *"Are the unresolved feelings or beliefs*

> *Holding onto anger is like you drinking cyanide and expecting someone else to die.*

*creating this stress really worth holding on to?"*

I came across an interesting article in an old Readers Digest. The article was written in 1987 and it was titled, "WARNING! DAILY HASSLES ARE HAZARDOUS"

> *University of Michigan sociologist Lois Verbrugge, who followed the daily lives of 589 men and women, found that daily irritations triggered bad moods, which, in turn, were followed by physical troubles.*

> *Studies among 210 Florida police officers showed that it wasn't the dramatic but relatively rare stress of apprehending criminals that caused distress. 'It was the accumulation of everyday hassles like too much paperwork,' reports Charles Speilberger, a psychologist at the University of South Florida.*

*Psychologist, Author Stone at the State of New York Stony Brook medical school found that minor daily stresses had increased three to five times before the onset of upper respiratory illnesses among a group of Long Island husbands.*

*In an earlier study Stone had 50 couples rate their daily experiences. The five most common hassles he found were conflicts with one's spouse, children or business colleagues, pressures at work and 'personal problems'. And he found that minor hassles were better predictors of illness rates than were major events from the past year. Brewing over arguments and misunderstandings from days, months and even years past were major stressors.*

Holding on to the disservices of your life will only manifest waning health. Joy will elude you and wealth will remain something foreign for others to attain....but not you, and I'm not just speaking tangible financial wealth.

All for the sake to "be right", your life will continue to *Research shows that 47% of all cancer is related to unresolved anger. Meanwhile, the other person has no frickin' idea how you feel!*

run off of the same old paradigms that have yet to deliver you the life of unadulterated Health Joy & Prosperity. Is it truly worth it?

I could have continued to blame my parents and everyone else for my problems and come up with excuse after excuse why my life was not working.

I could have continued on that road that was mapped out for me to be a single parent of multiple children, on welfare, uneducated, and just hopeless.

I could have chosen to stay a victim of what he said about me, what she did to me, what they put on me, blah, blah, blah. But to tell the truth, I just got goddamn tired of burning in my own personal hell.

I share this to impress upon you - YOU are the only one in harm's way of your anger and resentment. YOU are the only one holding on to the emotion, not anyone else. They have long moved on. YOUR emotions become embedded into the very cells of YOUR body, not theirs. YOUR feelings make YOU sick, not them. I have to share the following report that will amaze you.

*In W.A Chapman's book "Your Cosmic Destiny" in which he describes experiments in the psychology laboratory where human breath was examined, they found that hatred, anger and jealousy caused different colored condensates from human breath from calmness and contentment, which upon analysis contained deadly poisons.*

*The poison of a few minutes jealousy is enough to kill a guinea pig.*

*An hour of anger produces enough poison to kill 80 guinea pigs!*

*On the other hand, happy, loving peaceful emotions produce some of the most powerful healing chemicals known to mankind.*

Holding on to anger and resentment is like drinking poison and expecting someone else to die.

All healing is a release of the past. To become whole in health, joyful and successful, you absolutely MUST

*If you choose to hold on to all of your emotional garbage at least you know the difference.*

release your anger and resentments.

Everyone always does the best they can at that moment in time. Including you. Including me. It may not be the most enlightened moment in their life, but they are doing the best that they can with what tools they have to work with.

Those that you are angry with were acting out of their own conditioning from their past based in fear, but not in their true and higher self. Remember who your anger is harming. You can choose to forgive or you can choose to hold on. Choose to be right or choose to be healthy, happy and prosperous. Do you really need to be right about the situation?

When you release them from their deed you automatically release the anger, resentment and pain from yourself.

Before I consciously began my journey, I heard about Ms. Oprah Winfrey's story. How could anyone with the kind of colored past as what she has experienced become the "O"? Not only has she overcome hurdles of adversity, she has truly made a mark - on the world! I thought to myself (with all due respect) if someone like that can overcome and make a difference, why can't I?

### Breaking from the Herd
The birds of my feather knew there was something special / different about me. At the time, I just couldn't see my true self. I was dealing with – no, holding onto so much emotional garbage. Sometimes the slightest situation would set me off.

I had to raise my calibration. I began my quest and wanted so much for some of my friends and family to come with me, but they couldn't. They were happy and content "in their world", but I yearned for stimulation.

This was my journey and mine alone. The more I resisted my calling for change, it became a burden as my soul was crying out for freedom from the emotional hell I was living in.

I knew I could not do this alone. I needed a teacher, a

*If you can't change the people you hang around*

*Change the people you hang around.*

guide, a mentor. Although my friends for that time of my life were cool, they were much like me. They had a lot of their own emotional stuff to manage. I needed someone that would be able to share with me another way. A brighter way. I had to change my social circle and I did. Guidance from Gabriela opened a flood gate.

### EXERCISE II
Looking back at Exercise I, clearly these situations are hurtful, but now think for a minute. How will these affairs support your growth?

When you remove that false ego out of the way and really think this through, holding on to this stuff really does not support you or your growth at all. Actually, it hinders and even retards you from stepping into your greatness (and it can give you wrinkles).

Forgiveness of others is a daily walk. Forgiveness of yourself is an infinite walk.

How is holding on to these emotional ties benefiting you? When you think about these situations, how does it make you feel emotionally – sad, angry, anxious?

OK, now notice your body. How are you feeling in your body? Can you feel the tension across your shoulders, what about the temples of your head? Is your jaw tense? Now notice your chest (actually your heart). Does it feel tight? Whatever tension you are feeling in your muscles is the same tension your body is experiencing throughout.

Review Exercise I and pay careful attention to your physiology. Here in Exercise II check off the points of tension you feel as you go back to the memories of Exercise I.

☐ Head    ☐ Neck    ☐ Shoulders    ☐ Jaw

☐Neck    ☐ Chest    ☐ Stomach    ☐ Back

☐Hands    ☐ Knees    ☐Buttocks

Now notice the temperature of your body. Does the thought of these situations make you feel hot or cold?

Before we move on, I want you to take time out and just chill for a moment. Find a comfortable place to sit back and relax and take in deep diaphragm breaths. Again notice each and every muscle in your body. Where you feel tension, release, relax and let go.

Isn't it amazing, when you take notice, just how much control you really do have? This same peace you experience in your moment of relaxation is the same moment you can call forth at will. You dear heart, are the one in control.

This is a meditative prayer I share with my Creator.

*Mother Father God and all that is pure love and light, manifest through me abundant joy, ageless health, harmony and financial prosperity.*

*Thank you for my teachers and my lessons. You have a plan for me to step into my greatness to fulfill my ministry here on earth. You have designed me for leadership and I accept it fully.*

*Mother Father God, my heart of strife against _____, please remove this burden from me. Spring from within me the love and compassion to release and forgive them – just as you love and forgive me.*

*I know I have a calling on my life Mother Father God and I am thankful for my lessons.*

*Bless _____, that they too will step into the light of their greatness.*

*I release this all to you Mother Father God and now I am whole.*

*Thank you.*

# Chapter Five

## DESIRES OF THE HEART

I had to stop and ponder this for a moment. If only I could understand how to bring forth my desires, without cause for hesitation what would I choose?

I bought a journal and began writing these things out. Gabriela told me that if I take time to write my desires, it would become clear to me. If it's clear to me, then it would be clear to God as well!

I use to wonder why it seemed as though God wasn't listening to me, especially when I had been told that I would receive the desires of my heart. Well, I found out that it's kinda hard to receive the desires if I couldn't be clear on what my desires were.

Funny enough, when I had to sit down and commit my top five desires to paper, it took me about an hour to figure it out. First of all, I had so much chatter running through my mind. You know – coulda, shoulda, woulda.

I got into a quiet space. I turned off the television, lit a candle and some temple incense. There I sat – me, the silence, a flickering candle, burnt offering and my thoughts.

Once I dismissed the noise, I was able to focus.

The top five things I wanted most to experience were:

1. I wanted my physical, emotional and spiritual health to be whole.
2. I wanted to have a closer relationship with my daughter.
3. I wanted to be able to speak with my mother without feeling such intense anger and hostility.
4. I wanted a companion to talk to and grow with, sharing our lives together.
5. I wanted to experience overflowing financial success and help others do the same.

*It is written that God will give you the desires of your heart.*

*Are you clear about the desires of your heart? If not, how can you expect God to answer them?*

I can't begin to tell you what writing out my top five desires did for me. Just that simple exercise alone gave me so much clarity and from my clarity, things began to shift *dramatically* like you would not believe.

What are the top 5 things you most want to do, have, be or experience? Really, stop and think about this for a moment. Too often we wallow in what we don't have, and it seems to only attract to us more of -- WHAT WE DON'T HAVE!

*"I don't have the money to…", or "I can't afford to…"* or *I can't understand why so-n'-so…"*

These are all conversations of lack. So now that you are clear on what you don't want. Let's talk about what you do want!

That which is like unto itself attracts the same. Birds of a feather flock together. You are creating 24 hours a day, 7 days a week, however, mostly by default. The more you spin in what you don't want, the more it will keep coming to you, be it people, situations, or whatever!

Imagine what your life would be like to achieve all that you, not only need-- but want! What does that *feel* like? Close your eyes. Can you really see yourself living it? What does it *feel* like? Now, what is your "reason why"? Why do you desire this? Your reason why should put a fire in the pit of your belly. It should be that thing that wakes you up at 4:30 in the morning ready to get the day started so you can get that much closer to your goal.

Right now, you are tapping into that gift that I found in me. God's gift of the "hidden mystery". The hidden mystery is **you** dear heart!

Just like I tapped into my gift, in the silent room of just me, my thoughts, a flickering candle and temple incense smoke, you will tap into the Devine that is within you to call it forth.

## EXERCISE III

What are the top 5 desires of your heart?

Write them out. I promise you, once you are clear; **you will attract unto you what your heart truly desires.**

1. What is your desire?

   _____

   _____

   _____

   Why do you want this?

   _____

   _____

   _____

   _____

   _____

   How would you feel if you achieved your goal?

   _____

   _____

   _____

   _____

   _____

   _____

   How would you feel if you did not achieve your goal?

   _____

   _____

   _____

   _____

*How aimless to live this beautiful life and not have a dream to want to make manifest and a plan to make it happen.*

2. What is your desire?

_____
_____
_____

Why do you want this?

_____
_____
_____
_____
_____

How would you feel if you achieved your goal?

_____
_____
_____
_____
_____
_____

How would you feel if you did not achieve your goal?

_____
_____
_____
_____

3.  What is your desire?

    _____
    _____
    _____

    Why do you want this?

    _____
    _____
    _____
    _____
    _____

    How would you feel if you achieved your goal?

    _____
    _____
    _____
    _____
    _____
    _____

    How would you feel if you did not achieve your goal?

    _____
    _____
    _____
    _____

4.  What is your desire?

    _____
    _____
    _____

    Why do you want this?

    _____
    _____
    _____
    _____
    _____

    How would you feel if you achieved your goal?

    _____
    _____
    _____
    _____
    _____
    _____

    How would you feel if you did not achieve your goal?

    _____
    _____
    _____
    _____

5.  What is your desire?

    _____

    _____

    _____

    Why do you want this?

    _____

    _____

    _____

    _____

    _____

    How would you feel if you achieved your goal?

    _____

    _____

    _____

    _____

    _____

    _____

    How would you feel if you did not achieve your goal?

    _____

    _____

    _____

    _____

If you do not have enough emotion around your "reason why" it is not going to stick long enough to make a true change in your life.

What are you no longer willing to settle for? Really meditate on this.

*What would you set your intentions on if you were certain that you could not, would not fail?*

Do you know the following people?

## PERSON A

Mr. / Ms. Life is Great! They seem to have it all. Impermeable amounts of energy, great health, radiant personality, good looks, charm, all with a knack for having the Midas touch.

If you call them on the phone with drama, you may not get a whole lot of time because drama zaps them of their energy. They will quickly change the conversation to help you figure it out, or they will cut the call short, *"Girl, let me get off this phone. I got a million things to do!"* And you know what? They actually do have a million things to do. They are living their lives. They are living their desires!

Just being in their presence makes you feel like you could do anything. They see life as a game. A game worth winning!

They walk into a room and you can feel the energy just lift!

## PERSON B

Mr. / Ms. Schleprock. Not only is their health challenged, but that is all they talk about – how sick they have been, their last visit to the emergency room, and the latest drug their doctor has put them on this week.

A conversation on the telephone with them is exhausting. They are full of drama and always crying broke, and no I'm not just talking financially (although that is the typical conversation). They just seem to spin in broken dreams, broken promises, and their broken heart.

They walk into a room, and like a wet blanket, you can feel the barometric pressure of their dark heavy cloud of depression.

What makes Person A so different from Person B? Is it a secret? Is the difference found in their up-bringing, education, intelligence, skills, timing, work habits, contacts, luck, or their choice of businesses?

**The secret is…** *THERE IS NO SECRET!*

Person A just made a decision. When they close their eyes and visualize their desires, they write it down and then they take the necessary steps to make it all happen. And get this - it starts with their health!

> *"The outer conditions of a person's life will always be found to reflect their inner beliefs."*
> *- James Allen*

It's hard for me to believe that I use to be Person B. What in the heck was I thinking? Actually, that is part of the problem - I wasn't thinking. I was just going along with the status quo, being a herded sheep.

I could feel that I had something within me – something special. Everyone around me could see it, but at the time, I could not figure it out and because the friends I had around me were "at my same level" they couldn't direct me either. In order to make a change – in order for me to transform my life, I had to transform my habits. This included my associations.

Getting clear about my desires was a big step. From my desires, the next question that came to me was what do I want to contribute to the world? What could I offer that would impact not just one life, but many?

I knew that I was not living my life big enough. My life was living me. I was constantly giving away my power to everything and everyone else, and then holding them to blame.

As I was coming up through the ranks of corporate, I primarily just showed up so that I could get money to pay my bills. Now from the outside my career looked glamorous. My corporate background was marketing and I have held very high profile positions with major sports, entertainment and Wall Street financial firms. I have wined and dined with some of the world's top executives and even royalty.

When the night came to an end and I was left to trail home alone, it was there that the haunting of my inner
knowingness was telling me that my time and talents were not being utilized. I was literally wasting my life away.

In that present moment I couldn't see what else I was supposed to do. I mean heck, I had my apartment in NYC and my custom design clothes, and my pet, and my title and I had built this image. What was I suppose to do? I was stuck! At the time, I had no idea that I could chose differently. I felt like just another crab in the barrel. And I was.

*If you are not happy and healthy, or if you are missing your target of prosperity, it is likely you are attempting far too hard to be right (my way or the highway).*

*So tell me... how is that workin' for ya so far?*

As I began my work to unravel all the toxicity I had allowed my life to coil in, there came about a whole new purpose. This was by no way immediate. First and foremost, I had to take care of Madison.

It is my belief that we (especially women) often take up everyone else's cross including our own. We spend so much time trying to "measure up". To what? Expectations – expectations we put on ourselves, expectations we allow others to put on us, expectations of society, etc, etc, etc.

We are quick to come to the rescue of everyone else that calls for us, yet we won't rescue ourselves. It's our nature to nurture, but it should not be to the detriment of own needs.

I placed a lot of expectations on myself. I felt that I had to seeing that my mother really didn't expect much to come out of my life. I can recall being six years old and my mother telling me that she expected me to end up with a house full of babies by different men, uneducated and on welfare.

This was just one of many negative childhood replays I held on to and allowed it to spin a web of tangled emotions in the confines of my memories, bedding into my body.

> *There is nothing cute are sexy about giving from an empty cup. Give from your overflow. Take care of yourself FIRST! Trust me, everyone else will benefit greatly.*

As I became an adult, everything that my mother wanted to accomplish but did not, I set my intention on doing just that. I was driven by spite and revenge. I drove luxury foreign cars, I lived in the most affluent suburbia neighborhoods, I socialized with the who's who and my daughter went to the best schools in the state.

My daughter and I traveled, shopped, played, had pets, you name it. Anything I could do to one up on my

mother was the name of the game for me.
Funny… with all these one-ups, you would think
that I would be so proud of my
accomplishments, right?

### WRONG!

Instead, my life was a daily emotional
Amtrak train wreck.

> *You can be right or you can be happy, healthy and prosperous.*
>
> *You can be right or you can be depressed, sickly and broke.*

# Chapter Six

## THINK IT SPEAK IT BE IT

When I got my diagnosis and prognosis, I had to get real present with myself. I couldn't do anything about the past and at the time I had no idea about how to create my future. So, I figured I might as well work on this very moment. And then the next moment when it came, and then the next.

The most important thing to the conditioned mind is to be right.

Like most, I was run by my painful past circumstances. The past was affecting not only who I was at the moment of that time, it was also affecting my health. I was dragging that old baggage into my current and future relationships over and over again and it was wearing on me like a cheap suit.

Our thoughts and words are so extremely powerful! In the beginning

*Stick and Stones may break my bones but words will never hurt me. What a CROCK! EVERY WORK HAS A VIBRATORY ENERGY; therefore it has POWER!*

was the word. We have learned from biblical stories that God spoke and the Earth was formed. Words are POWERFUL!

The words we use, use us. We can speak life, health, healing, joy, love, and prosperity into our life just as we can speak sickness, fatigue *("I'm sick and tired of...")*, sadness, loneliness *("I can do bad all by myself")* and financial destitute *("I'm broke. I don't have the money to...")* into our life.

Be mindful of what you are claiming into your life as well. If you are consistently claiming your physical, emotional and fiscal situations, your mind and body are receiving it as so.

By saying, *"my cancer"*, *"my high blood pressure"*, *"my diabetes"*, *"my bad skin"*, *"my broken heart"*, *"my strained relationship"*, *"my debts"*, etc. you are claiming all of this into your life as so. Instead, refer to the challenge you are experiencing as, *"**the** cancer"*, *"**the** high blood pressure"*, *"**the** debts"*.

Whenever I find myself getting caught up in my own spin and speaking claim to something I know is not serving me, I energetically cancel it out by saying,

***Cancel, cancel and purify
through the power of love.***

Two of the most powerful combination of words are - *I AM*. God spoke and said, *"I AM that I AM"*. This I share with you – be exceptionally prudent, aware and mindful when speaking, *"I AM _____."*

***What you think and feel so shall you manifest. What you speak so shall it BE!***

| Disempowering | Empowering |
| --- | --- |
| *I'm*<br>*Unworthy, undeserving* | *I AM*<br>*Worthy and Deserving of love, health, joy and prosperity.* |
| *I'm*<br>*Sick and Tired of....* | *I AM*<br>*Mindful that this lesson is coming to me again for a reason.* |
| *I'm*<br>*Broke / Poor to keep me humble and close to God* | *I AM*<br>*Worthy of wealth and success and I stand humbly grateful for all my blessings.* |
| *I'm Not...* | *I AM...* |

### Speak Powerfully
### That What You Intend to Create!

What I have learned is that life is scientifically systematic. Everything happens in decency and order. Joy, health and then prosperity.

Oh sure, you will find many instances where there are financially wealthy people, but if you truly pay attention, like Dr. Mya Angelou says, "People will tell / show you exactly where they are. When they do, believe them."

My friend once shared something so powerful with me during one of our morning conversations. He said, *"What goes on behind closed eyes is vastly different from what goes on behind closed doors."* What we do consciously behind closed doors eventually comes to light. What we do unconsciously (blindly) is still played out in the darkness of our ignorance.

The ultimate in this life is to have it ALL – Health, Happiness and Prosperity and to have it all more abundantly!

Even in health, healing and anti-aging, there is a system to maximize diet, treatments and supplements. It would be senseless to take supplements if your body is not able to process them. It would be like throwing pearls to swine to cleanse and then go to Fat Burger and load up on burgers n' fries and a milkshake. Oh, and don't forget to top it off with a diet soda.

Like the proverbial light bulb coming on, I finally got it. Once I got it, I began focusing on regaining my health - systematically. As my well-being came into balance, I began to feel better about my life and it

showed in my body. I beam with youth and vitality. Once I recognized my joy, my productivity picked up and now prosperity flows as my cup runnith over.

If any of this resonates with you, then please dedicate your time to study the message delivered in this book with an open mind and heart. It may very well be the most important information you will read and yet, this is just the beginning. That which suits you, take it and hold on to it. That which doesn't suit you leave it behind.

In the next index of this book I am sharing with you my interpretations of the natural alternative therapies I have used personally to regain my health from cervical cancer.

I have also included my current routine of anti-aging therapies, supplements and nutriceuticals I use on an ongoing bases to maintain my health and youthful vitality.

Anti-aging begins from the inside out, not the outside in. Anti- acne topical creams, liposuction, and body shapers may support maintenance, but if you want REAL transformation, if you want to seize the fountain of youth – start within!

I am not a professional of conventional medicine. What I am sharing with you is solely my personal testimony of what has worked for me. I would strongly suggest you seek advice from a wellness professional or your medical physician on how to process forward with any health and wellness regimen.

Thank you for allowing me to share my story with you. I hope there is something in my experiences that will help you to understand, you are not alone.

God is setting you up for a breakthrough. Are you ready?

*According to Buckminster Fuller, there is a tendency for all living things to increasingly achieve higher and higher levels of energetic output and consequently transform. However, so many are living a tendency to reach lower and lower levels of energetic output until eventually there is failure.*

*N O T E:*
*FAILURE IS NOT AN OPTION HERE!*

# INDEX II
# Chapter Seven

## AN ALGORITYM FOR HEALING

*There are genocidal disasters happening daily to our physical health, emotional stability and financial well-being. Unless we grasp the truth of overstanding that we are the magnificent manifestors of our circumstances, we will forever remain in captivity of the disturbed creation of our ignorance.*

*-Madison Carlista*

What we do consciously behind closed doors eventually comes to light. What we do unconsciously (blindly) is still played out in the darkness of our ignorance.

What I have come to understand isn't a huge mystery, at least not anymore. For centuries, the very same principles that I will share with you were once shrouded in obscurity. Over time we (you and me and ages of recent past) have paid dearly for our ignorance.

There is an algorithm to health and that system is most easily influenced when all six of the body's sense faculties are employed. The sense of sight, sound, taste, audio, touch and spirit.

There is an algorithm to sickness and disease. It is very systematic. If you or a loved one are dealing with heath issues, note the function or ill-function of your senses. I am certain you will note that your sense faculties are either very dull and waning, or mute. This did not just happen overnight.

All of your senses are stimulated by your environment. If your environment is polluted, tense and dark, so will your body respond in kind as you can only take on and become a product of such. If your environment is clean, relaxing and bright so will your body respond in kind as you can only take on and become a product of such.

When I was going through my health rehabilitation, one of the first things I did was reset my home environment. Your home is your sanctuary and no matter what is going on outside your doors, it is your home where you will find refuge for peace, joy, healing and prosperity.

First thing I did to change my environment was open my shades to let in natural light. I was affected by S.A.D (Seasonal Affective Disorder) also known as winter depression. For me, the lack of sunlight could set heavy moods of depression that sort of loomed over me.

Another thing, I disconnected the cable and sold my 60" flat screen television. The reason I got rid of my television is because the influence the media has on the human psyche. There is so much negative feedback on television. Let's take the news. Before you can get 10 minutes into the evening news you will hear about death, destruction, war, and the economic crisis. All this mess is enough to send your heart racing and elevate your blood pressure to a boiling point. The media can actually control your emotions!

I got rid of my microwave. Microwaves actually breaks down the molecular structure of food (and water) rendering it void of any nutrients. Why do you think parts of Europe have bans against microwave cooking? I read a fascinating report by Dr. Hans Ulrich Hertel that noted the health risks of food prepared in a microwave vs. food prepared in a conventional oven. Definitely take time to read up on Dr. Hertel and his report.

Everything chemical that I could afford to replace in my home I did. EVERYTHING I put on or in my body was immediately exchanged for natural / organic products. I went to Whole Foods market and got my toothpaste, shampoo and conditioner, hair oil, body oil, soap and mouthwash.

What I have learned about the chemicals in our daily products is staggering. *The Cure for All Cancers* by Dr. Hulda Clark is like my bible for all day to day products that are chemically harmful. The things we take for granted can grant us a one way ticket to all myriads of sickness and dis-ease, if we don't take the time to learn. Learn how to care for your health and then effectively apply that which has been learned.

I redesigned my home by moving my furniture around and got rid of all the clutter. Just by opening and clearing my space, I was able to generate a flow of energy that felt very open and free. Everything I did for the inside of my body, I worked just as deliberately for my outer environment to reflect the transformation.

During one of my coaching sessions with another one my spiritual mentors, Ma'at Seba, I was gifted a small collection of temple incense to burn. Now when I first received this gift, I didn't take it seriously. I figured it was just some sticks and cones of "flavored smoke". Not at all - the incense and oils I was given were temple incense and specifically prepared for stimulating a vibration for healing.

There is a whole sacred science behind incense. Much of the commercial incense is full of animal dung fillers and oils cut with chemicals to stretch the production. Breathing the fumes from the smoke of some of the cheap store bought incense can cause additional stress on the immune system.

My marvel of these curious smokes lead me to study aromatherapy and the healing and calming benefits. Conventional medicine will argue that aromatherapy provides no advantage to healing, but they do support the fact that our sense of smell can influence calm or calamity. If aromatherapy can invoke calm, wouldn't it make sense that the calming nature can support healing? Duh!

There was an algorithm I used to get myself into the situation I was facing with my health. Whether I was conscious of it or not, I still produced an outcome and the cause of my lifestyle produced an effect.

That's all life is, cause and effect. In my analysis, if I was smart enough to get myself into this quagmire unconsciously, then I was going to study to consciously understand how to get myself out of this mess.

Anyone…. everyone has access to infinite health, inner peace and joy, and unlimited wealth, but I will tell you, if you don't take time to understand the science of life – the science of health, you will forever remain a captive of your own ignorance.

There is a study that claims ill-health, obesity and dis-ease are all products of poverty. I half heartedly agree; I say it is a product of not only economics, but ignorance as well. It is so systematically set up for the slaughter of the weak that the fallout is yet to be realized.

I know a lot of very wealthy people; some are even dear friends of mine. They travel the world over, broker million dollar deals, indulge in the finest food, drink and yes, recreational substances the world has to offer, damn near every day. To the undiscerning spirit it looks like they have the world on a string. They are living the life! In my ignorance, this is what I too thought. I thought they were living the life. Heck, I was out there too trying to live it with them and I did so on many occasions.

Each time I was out "living life" my body was giving me subtle hints that this was taxing my health. In the darkness of my ignorance, I continued to overlook the signs, but each time the message my body was sending got more and more severe.

It started with the headaches, constipation, gas, bloating and indigestion. I could go days without having a bowel movement. Another thing I remember was that I seem to be constantly clearing my throat or coughing up mucus. My body was so full of mucus that my eyes would constantly drain. There were so many signs that my body was out of balance. Following is list of the other challenges I had to deal with:

- Halitosis
- Vaginal Discharge / Yeast Infections
- Skin Breakouts (especially on my buttocks, back thighs, and back arms)
- Dry / Flaking Skin

- Blurred Vision
- Heavy Menses
- Bloating and Gas
- Ringing in the Ears
- Spotting Between Menses
- Bleeding During Sex (this totally freaks guys out)
- Uncomfortable / Painful sex
- Mood Swings
- Headaches
- Fatigue So Bad I Could Hardly Function
- Mucus Drain from Inner Corner of My Eyes
- Constantly Clearing My Throat from Phlegm
- Itchy Nose, Ears and Rectum (sign of parasites)
- And when I did have bowel movements, it would be like little hard rabbit pellets.

Little did I know at the time, I was literally decaying, slowly, but none the less decaying from the inside out. My depleted energy was a clear indication that my lifestyle was smoldering out my life force.

To digress a bit, I did get a second opinion. I heard about a cervical cancer analysis that was much more on point than the pap smear exam. Pap smear testing is only about 60% - 70% accurate. The cervical cancer test has an accuracy of 100% as it actually measures the blood. The blood will always tell the truth.

With a cervical cancer test, a healthy woman would measure between 500 – 700. Cervical cancer would measure from about 1170 on up. My results came back with a rating of 1350.

I made the decision that I would only tell a select handful of people about my challenge. The people I shared my secret with are prayer warriors with a "failure is not an option" mentality.

My friends and family mean well, but not all of them are aware of their own power. People will cry and talk you into your own grave, if you listen to them. Last thing I needed was someone laying me to rest with their "poor Madison" conversation. Therefore, I chose people that would speak, pray, meditate and see life in me.

Now, let's move forward. I called a very dear friend of mine. She is a medical doctor as well as a doctor of naturopathic medicine. I went by her office and took all of my notes and files. I made it very clear to Dr. Sharon "O" that I was not going to do the surgery nor was I going glow in the dark from radiation. My friend looked at me, smirked and shook her head. *"All right, very well. We have work to do."*

Dr. O put together a plan that looked like a strategy for battle. After we charted everything out Sharon said, "*I want you to work with a spiritual mentor.*" She gave me name of a woman named Ma'at Seba. I couldn't understand what a spiritual mentor had to do with my healing, but for where I was, I allowed myself to be open.

I took my schedule of fasts, therapies and supplements prescribed by my naturopathic, MD. As I was about to walk out of her office, Dr. "O" stopped me. "*Madison, you may not understand what I am about to say to you, but in time, you will.*" I looked at Sharon with baited breath hoping she was not going to deliver me more bad news. "*Madison, what you have been given is a gift. Like I said, right now you may not understand it, but in time, you will.*" It was everything I could do to keep from slicing Sharon up one way and back down the other. "*A Gift!*" I scoffed. "*Yeah, right. You're right, I don't understand.*" I kept my final thoughts to myself, but gave her a look that said it all as I walked out the door with my mission in hand.

The first order of business was to drastically change my diet. It became my understanding that so much of sickness and dis-ease begins and ends with our diets. So many of our foods are literally cooked to devitalization and death and my diet was for crap, truth be told. Probably 70% of my intake came out of a box, can or restaurant menu.

I went on a 45 day fresh squeezed greens juice and alkaline water fast and prepared myself for a series of colon hydrotherapy treatments.

The body uses its most energy in digesting food. By doing my fresh organic fruits and veggies in juice form, I was able to nourish my body and use the reserved energy to heal.

My cousin GiBi told me about an exotic fruit from South America that had tremendous healing properties and was high in anti-oxidants. She ordered my first case and gifted it to me. As I was looking over my wellness strategy from Sharon, I saw her notes on anti-oxidants.

I sat down and over the next couple of days put together my schedule in correlation to Dr. O's nutritional and cleansing recommendations.

Daily Schedule of Food & Supplement Intake:
- ✓ Bottle of mangosteen juice drunken throughout the day.
- ✓ 6- 8 oz glasses of fresh squeezed greens juice with ½ tsp cayenne pepper per glass throughout the day.
- ✓ 60 oz of alkaline water throughout the day.
- ✓ 2- 6 oz servings of Essiac tea
- ✓ 2 probiotic capsules in the PM.
- ✓ 2 omega fish oil caps in the AM.
- ✓ 4 fiber caps in the AM & PM.

- ✓ 2 digestive enzymes in the AM & PM.
- ✓ 2 Tsp of liquid CalMag before bedtime
- ✓ 2 capsules of black walnut / wormwood / cloves parasite cleanse before bedtime.

Weekly Schedule of Therapies:
- ✓ Colon Hydrotherapy 3x / week.
- ✓ Hot Epsom Salt Water Soak Baths 2x/week.
- ✓ Hydrogen Peroxide Bath Soaks (pint added) 2x/week.
- ✓ Ionic Cleanse 3x / week.
- ✓ Hyperbaric Chamber 1x / week.
- ✓ Lymphatic Massage or Endermologie 1x / week.
- ✓ Derma Detoxification 1x / month.
- ✓ FIR Sauna 1x / week.
- ✓ Coaching w/ Spiritual Mentor 2x / week.

Daily Practices to Raise My Energetic Immunity
- ✓ Wearing My Compression Garment for Lymphatic Stimulation
- ✓ Exercise to Increase Oxygen Flow
- ✓ Burnt Offering (temple incense)
- ✓ Prayer
- ✓ Journaling
- ✓ Meditation
- ✓ Reading

This was my schedule at a glance. My schedule was broken down by times, intake, practices and so on. I kept a very detailed daily log of intake, elimination, activities and everything.

The first week or two was slow going, but I did not give up. My *reason why* is what kept me pushing, even during those days of impatience when I felt like my work was futile.

After the first 30 days, the change was amazing! I could feel the difference in my energy (internal), and then people began to comment on my skin, my eyes and just my appearance in general (external). I still had a lot of work to do, but I was getting my glow back!

Every 30 days I did a live blood cell analysis to monitor my progress.

# Chapter Eight

## FOOD – THE FAST & FURIOUS

The fast was most challenging the first couple of days. I had never done an intentional fast before. Oh sure, I had gone all day and forgotten to eat because my schedule got so hectic, but never had I fast on nothing but liquids.

The first two to three days I could have eaten a bear! OMG! I kept my focus on my *reason why*. During this time my daughter was living with her father, and she was my main reason why I moved forward with laser sharp intention.

The reason for the fast was to give my body a rest. The body utilizes its most energy in digesting food. During a liquid fast, the body is still getting all the nutrients needed, but it doesn't have to exert as much energy to break everything down. The nutrients from the liquids are immediately distributed throughout the organs.

There was a great deal to learn about fasting. There was a great deal to learn about food. All fasts are not equal, neither is all food. Much of the reason for my health challenges had a great deal to do with my diet. Prior to this instantaneous transformation, my diet was loaded with processed foods, fast foods, junk foods and sweetened drinks.

Looking back, my dietary habits go back to my parents. My mother was not much of a cook, so I can clearly recall eating a lot of TV dinners, can spaghetti, boxed macaroni and cheese or packaged meats. If anything was cooked, it was fried to a second death by lard.

I was Daddy's Punkin. I never wanted or needed for anything. Before I came to live with him at nine years old he was a true to life bachelor. Growing up with Daddy, Burger King was a staple in our diet. For me, Whopper with cheese and all the dressings. I did not care for pickles, but I did like the taste it infused into my burger. I would also order a large fry and Dr. Pepper. If it wasn't Burger King, it was a Big Mac from McDonald's with a large French fry and chocolate shake. The main food staples in our home consisted of pork skins, Snicker bars, Oreo cookies, Raisin Bran, Whole Vitamin D milk, Lipton sweet tea powder mix, packaged lunch meat and white bread.

As I look back over my life with my mom and with my dad (they separated before I was a year old) I don't recall either one of them ever having a piece of fresh fruit or vegetable in the house. So much of our diet consisted of processed foods and fast foods.

When we did have home cooked meals during the holidays, Sunday dinners, or other family gatherings, much of the food was fried, heavily seasoned with salt (with even more salt added on the plate) or sugar, and the vegetables were cooked to death – just no life force left in them at all. Don't get me wrong, the food was delicious! Chil' my family can put a good foot in some home cookin', but to eat like that consistently as a lifestyle is what was so harmful.

You see, it wasn't so much that I got cancer because of my family's health history. What happened is that I carried on these habits and eating practices from my childhood through my adolescence and into my adult life. It is here that the sins of the parents are passed down to the child – through HABITS – not heredity.

I had maintained the same eating habits and lifestyle practices for more than 30 years of my life. In my family, no one spoke of cleansing or exercise. No one even mentioned drinking water. As I look back with the understanding I have now, I am certain that many of my family members dealt with numerous digestive and elimination issues, allergies, joint pains and other ailments.

My family, on both my mother's side and my father's side are very astute. My mother's side of the family have entrepreneurial spirits. My father's side of the family are educators. Many of my relatives on both sides of my parents are and have been very active in the community and church. These people are the salt of the earth, and yet still without understanding of health.

This unknowingness is not just within my family, I see it across the board in many families – very affluent families – so conventional education has absolutely nothing to do with this particular lack of knowledge. It's just an understanding that is not mainstream, yet.

It also baffles me how many faith based organizations do not adhere to the principals of health and healing. Saved, sanctified and full of cancer, diabetes, high blood pressure, you name it. How can a leader stand in front of his / her followers and not teach the biblical principles of health? I guess that can be a challenge when the preacher is loaded up on diabetic and high blood pressure medicine and just a lard fried chicken drumstick from a heart attack. I mention this with all due respect - truly. Hmmm, I see I have gotten a bit off topic. I digress.

Once I began to eliminate a lot of the old dietary teachings I noticed a huge shift. I have had digestive problems since I can remember. I can clearly recall being five years old and my mother giving me a suppository because my bowels had not moved in days.

After the first 3 days of my fast I had my first bowel movement - on my own! No laxatives, no prune juice, just the alkaline water and fresh squeezed liquid vegetable diet I had taken on.. This was a BIG deal for me. Although I was juicing everything, I was taking the fiber, enzymes and other supplements, so this encouraged much needed hydration and stimulated my system to process everything out of my body.

When I was not on a liquid fast, my diet (which is now a consistent lifestyle choice for me), is still very regimen. I resolved to eat mainly uncooked vegetables, fruits and raw nuts. Grains are a minor portion of my diet. When I do eat cooked foods, I include complex carbohydrates, like sweet potatoes squash, lima beans, lentils, and black beans. Simple carbohydrates and refined grains (like white sugar, high fructose corn syrup, white flour, pasta, macaroni, white potatoes, white rice and dairy products) are kept at a distant minimum. It has been my experience and from all of my reading and research that the body easily converts simple carbohydrates into glucose, and this glucose provides cancer cells their main source of energy. In other words, this is what feeds cancer!

I abstain from animal protein. When animal flesh is cooked and eaten, it makes the body more acidic creating a cancer friendly environment. There is also a huge demand placed on the pancreas, that is already challenged from the lack of nutritional support. The pancreas is responsible for producing the digestive enzymes necessary for digesting Lambert, Millie the Cow, and ol' Kentucky the Frying Chicken.

Other foods that will not kiss my lips are soy oil, corn oil, and other polyunsaturated and hydrogenated oils, including margarine, aspartame (i.e. Nutri-Sweet, Equal and diet sodas), chemical preservatives, coffee, food dyes, and alcohol. These foods make my body encourage cancer growth.

Today I eat a lot of what is called, Super Foods that greatly support my immune system. My diet consists of garlic (1-2 cloves a day), deep green leafy veggies (collards, kale, turnip greens), especially juiced as they are rich sources of magnesium, very alkalizing and oxygen rich. I love pineapple, pomegranates, raspberries, figs, blackberries, blueberries and persimmons. They are all rich in anti-oxidants. Papaya and the seeds have a very high protein digesting enzyme value. I also eat a lot of sprouted beans like lima beans and black eye peas. Soy bean sprouts are a complete source of easily digestible protein, supporting higher alkalinity.

Now, you're likely not going to find any government clinical studies that prove the effectiveness of the so called "Super Foods". Reason why is because there is no profit to be gained from the FDA (Food and Drug Administration) and AMA (American Medical Association). You see, natural foods that grow from the earth cannot be patented, so there is no monetary motivation for them to bankroll expensive studies.

Be aware, be very aware. The government has been trying for years to find its way around this. One step they took was creating GMO (Genetically Modified Food). GMO was created all in the name of protecting the American public from contaminated foods. Remember the big scare back in the summer of 2008 with spinach? What about the tomatoes? The spin on the story was that because of "human error" there is a need to create fruits and vegetables that are hardy enough to survive contamination. Because the American public is so asleep and gullible, we are being bamboozled into this belief. Thank God for the environmentalist groups that are keeping a watchful eye on the midnight congress sessions that try to pass bills limiting our access to natural foods and supplements.

If you want to get an ear and eyeful of information on this, go to YouTube and type in Codex Alimentarius.

# Chapter Nine

## THE S²O of H²O

Next to the air we breathe, water is the most powerful and necessary element of life and so many people have no idea the power water holds. Water alone has the power to heal, especially when you know how to recognize and use it adroitly.

In this new age of health awareness, we are spending over $80 billion a year on nutritional supplements, herbs, homeopathics, and the like. It has become common for a client / patient to leave the doctor's or health practitioner's office with a nutritional formulation in hand as part of a particular therapy.

It is amazing how so much time and money is being spent on supplements, organic foods, and natural remedies (some of which are very subtle and delicate) but little attention is given to the quality and effect of the water with which those items are taken. Then too, I have watched people knock back a whole handful of pills and/or supplements with a soda or milk. Now that move just baffles the hell out of me!

There are thousands of studies that speak on the water quality crisis and shortage. Depending on where you live, a simple water test would easily find trace amounts of nitrates, pesticides, heavy metals, radioactive compounds, petrochemicals, parasites, and drugs.

I wish here I could tell you to have no worries, our government is looking out for us. Well, like the saying goes, "The road to hell is paved with good intentions." In an effort to "clean" our waters, chlorine – a powerful disinfectant is used in virtually all public water supplies in America. The US Counsel on Environmental Quality has reported that individuals who drink and bath in chlorinated waters (which includes better than 90% of the population) have a 93% greater likelihood of getting cancer in their lifetime.

In January 2000, Sixty Minutes, the investigative TV program reported that as many as 100 million Americans were drinking water contaminated with MTBE, a gasoline additive that has been leaching into our water supplies since 1992. MTBE is believed to cause cancer in concentration as low as 10 parts per billion and unfortunately local water companies are helpless to remove it. Hence, the dawning of bottled water, yet there is still no assurance of safety. The problem is that the average consumer and even most medical professionals do not know what is the best way to treat water or the best source of water to drink.

Approximately 75% of your our body weight is water and water makes up over 80% of our brain and 90% of our blood. Since water is an integral part of every function of the body, there is now evidence to indicate that insufficient hydration of the body can, in itself, lead to or exacerbate specific health conditions and illnesses.

Quality hydration, particularly from alkaline water has been reported to reverse and minimize such conditions as premature aging, arthritis, heartburn, back pain, asthma, hypertension, constipation and migraine headaches, just to mention a few. In addition, alkaline water has been tremendously shown to have the following benefits:

- Alkaline water is better at helping the body absorb and assimilate nutrients into the blood stream and internal organs.
- Sufficient intake of clean water has been shown to cut the risk of certain cancers like colon, breast, bladder and kidney.
- Drinking alkaline water before meals helps with weight loss and weight control since it aids in digestion and reduces cravings.
- Water lubricates joints and muscles, reduces inflammation, aides in the recovery of injuries and decreases the risk of certain types of physical injuries like sprains and pulls.
- Proper hydration helps the body resist the formation of kidney stones, urinary tract infections and constipation. Water also accelerates the excretion of toxic waste from the body.

- As little as 2% dehydration can lead to significant short-term memory loss. Because alkaline water is actually absorbed into the cells of the body including the brain, mental performance is actually boosted.

The dilemma is to find the "perfect water". I have tried distilled water and reverse osmosis water, thinking the purest is the best. I have also used natural spring water, and even "designer" water. Although some of these waters are good, they each have their drawbacks.

It was not until I started drinking alkaline water that I truly noticed a huge shift in how my body was processing. This is only the half of it. Drinking alkaline water paired with my supplement intake was like a magnification of everything to the *inth* power!

Seeing what the water was doing to my body by drinking it, of course you know I had to take it to a whole new level. Yep, I took it there - douching and enemas.

Douching with alkaline water can help with reducing vaginal odor and yeast accumulation.

Preparing my enemas and home colonic treatments with alkaline water has proven to be extremely beneficial! I feel it helps my body to come into pH balance overall as there are nerves in the colon that correlate to every organ in the body. I'm telling you, if you have a headache, go clean your colon!

Do your research. All water is not created equally. So much is gained by its consumption and yet there are tremendous risks of contamination. If you log onto my site, you will see a video where I did a test of various bottled waters, facet water and a bottle of 7-up. All I can say… Eye Opening! Check it out www.madisoncarlista.com.

# Chapter Ten

## A SUPPLEMENT FOR SEXY
### The Importance of Fiber

<u>Soluble Fiber</u> soaks up cholesterol in the intestines and prevents it from being absorbed, eventually carrying it out of the body. Your body miraculously recognizes this decrease of cholesterol in the intestinal tract and responds by pulling cholesterol out of the bloodstream to replace the cholesterol that was removed from the intestines. As a result, the amount of cholesterol in the bloodstream goes down and so does the risk of heart dis-ease!

<u>Insoluble Fiber</u> acts like a scrub brush for the digestive tract. It tends to clump up in the digestive tract, and because it is not broken down and stays in solid form, it helps produce well sized stool and it also helps to retain water. This is why it is important to maintain proper water intake when taking fiber supplements.

So while soluble fiber is spongy, insoluble fiber is more coarse. The two together really help to cleanse the intestinal tract and push waste on through and out.

**Anti-Oxidants**

Anti-oxidants, with the new surgence of super fruits we are hearing this word thrown around like a hot potato. What is an anti-oxidant and why do we need them? Anti-oxidants inhibit unstable molecules know as free radicals. Free radical damage has been documented to lead to cancer.

Ok, so what is a free radical? Leave a bicycle outside for a year, what happens? The weather elements will break down the metal and cause it to rust. Toss a penny in a pond and over a period of time you will see that the water will turn the copper green. The oxygen in the water is breaking down the metal elements of the penny. Take an apple, slice it in half. You will notice that after just a few moments the flesh of the apple begins to turn brown. The apple is actually dying. Free radicals damage in the body is known as oxidative stress and plays a significant role in aging and cell damage. The same air that is decomposing the apple and breaking down the metal is the same air we are breathing. If the air we breathe is doing all this to food and metal, what is happening to our bodies? Got ya thinking now, right?

Free radicals and the damage they can do at the cellular level have received a lot of attention in the last few years. The oxidative stress caused by free radicals – which are produced during normal metabolism and cell function, as well as pollutants in our air, water and food – is implicated in everything from aging and wrinkling of skin to DNA damage, diabetes cancer and heart dis-ease. Our bodies age or decay over time due to free radicals which cause them to oxidize or "rust". This is clearly an issue for anyone concerned about their health, or just looking and feeling younger.

Anti-oxidants slow down the rate of cell aging and eliminate free radicals in the body. Naturally, anti-oxidants should be received through a balanced diet of alkalizing water, fruits, vegetables and grains, but because our soils are so depleted of nutrients due to all of the toxicity we bury in our grounds, dump in our waters and release in the air, our food supply is devitalized. It is best to get your anti-oxidants through a supplement, ideally liquid so that it can quickly and easily assimilate into the bloodstream.

Anti-oxidants neutralize free radicals as the natural by-product of normal cell processes. Cells become dis-eased because of the aging process. The cells age because they are taking in and holding on to waste that is robbing them of their vitality. With the cells holding on to the toxicity it causes a break down and dis-ease sets in.

Most anti-oxidants rally around each cell to protect them, and there are some anti-oxidants that actually penetrate the cells and extract the waste, depositing it back into the elimination channels to process out of the body.

When I was going through my transformation, I was drinking mangosteen juice like it was going out of style. I drank a bottle of it every day. At the time, mangosteen was the most potent anti-oxidant on the market I knew of. I can recall that after the first couple of days, I did notice a huge difference in my energy, primarily because my body was eliminating more.

There are a lot of wonderful concentrated anti-oxidant juices on the market: Noni, Gogi, Mangosteen, Pomegranate, Acai, and more. The only challenge I have about concentrates is that there is more sugar in these juices than what I would want to put in my body, but nonetheless, these juice drinks are still very powerful and have the highest ORAC value available individually.

Two of the best anti-oxidant juice supplements I have come across are extracts. One contains the top seven berries…all in one bottle! The other contains five berries, again all in one bottle! For an anti-oxidant addict like myself this is the Holy Grail! One juice is LeVive by Ardyss International. This juice has Gogi, Noni, Mangosteen, Pomerganent and Acai.

The other juice is eXfuse, which has Gac, Acai, Gogi, Noni, Fucoidan, Mangosteen and Seabuckthron. Both eXfuse and LeVive are powerful and when taken consistently with a clean balanced diet, the experience is transformative.

In Section III you will find a chart that lists these berries and what they are known to support.

**ORAC**

A lot of these new wonder juices that are coming out on the market boast about their ORAC value and how high theirs is in comparison to the other guys. Like "anti-oxidant" it is another really big word that has an important meaning, but very few know just what the heck it means, but is sounds great in a sentence and makes you come across really smart. Well, not here folks, here is where we walk our talk.

So, what is an ORAC? It stands for Oxygen Radical Absorbance Capacity. He who has the highest ORAC value wins. This system was developed by Dr. Guohua Coa, a chemist and physician with the National Institute of Aging. ORAC is just a fancy way of saying, *"How well does a certain food help my body fight dis-eases like cancer and diabetes, and keep me from aging."*

It has been well documented that foods with a high ORAC score have been able to protect cells and tissue from oxidative damage, reversing aging and dis-ease.

**CalMag (Calcium & Magnesium Liquid)**

<u>Calcium</u> makes your heart and other muscles contract. Magnesium makes your heart and other

muscles relax. Calcium is the most abundant mineral in your body. It is responsible for so many of the body's functions. Calcium is a key component for collagen. Collagen is the most abundant protein in your body and it works hand in hand with elastin, which supports the body's tissues. A tell-tell sign of a lack of calcium is in the skin. As you age, collagen degeneration can occur leading to wrinkles. If it's showing visible effects on your skin, then you can be sure it is also occurring under your skin in the bones, muscles and organs.

Magnesium deficiency can result in irregular heartbeats. If your heart beats too fast or too slow or it races, these are all typical signs of magnesium deficiency. Have you ever had a muscle cramp, like the ones that will clench your calf muscle like a vice grip in the still of the night when you are getting that really good sleep and will cause you to stand straight up on your mattress and contort like a pretzel as you try to massage it out? This is typical of magnesium deficiency. If this can happen to your calf muscle, then know that the same can happen to any other muscle or organ in your body.

Magnesium is very helpful in providing relief from constipation. High amounts of magnesium have always been found to bring relief. In fact, the only time when water-soluble magnesium does not relieve constipation is when enough is not taken. Unlike laxatives, magnesium will not irritate and break down the colon lining. Do keep in mind however that this is merely a quick fix and the cause of the system not flushing needs to be addressed properly.

Calcium and Magnesium work like hand in glove and it has been my experience that liquid assimilates easier into the body than pills.

## Omega Oils

Omega Oils, also known as EFA (Essential Fatty Acids) are healthy fats and have tons of health benefits, they include omega-3, omega-6, and omega-9. These EFAs provide support for numerous body functions. I have broken down each EFA and listed their benefits:

Omega 3 improves arthritis, reduces hypertension and risk of stroke, improves heart health, improves symptoms of Lupus, reduce depression and symptoms of other mental health problems, aid in colon cancer prevention, aid in preventing breast cancer, and supports weight loss by helping to control blood sugar levels.

Omega 6 reduces joint inflammation of rheumatoid arthritis, relieves symptoms of PMS, reduces symptoms of endometriosis and fibrocystic breasts, clear acne and other skin breakouts, enhance growth of healthy hair, nails and skin.

Omega 9 improves blood sugar maintenance and insulin resistance, protects and supports the immune system, reduces blood pressure and the risk of strokes.

**Digestive Enzymes**

The body naturally produces    but over a period of time and with improper diet our enzymes deplete. Digestive enzymes help your body to break down and absorb the foods you are eating and help to clean the blood. Lack of enzymes coupled with poor eating habits and poor digestion can lead to an overgrowth of yeast, parasites, food allergies, constipation, indigestion, gas and bloating leading to a myriad of more severe health issues.

A lot of enzymes are lost in cooking. Fire actually breaks down and depletes fruits and vegetables almost to nothing. The best way to retain the enzymatic value of your fresh organic produce is to prepare and eat it raw. You can get very creative with raw foods. There is more to raw food preparation than just salads you know? Do an online search or check out your neighborhood bookstore. Even, check out your closest Whole Foods market.

One of the best ways to help the body rebuild enzymes is to eat raw organic foods as much as possible. Any kind of heat treatment on foods destroys 100% of the enzymes.

Research suggests that eating cooked foods depletes the body's enzyme potential, and robes the body of energy needed for growth, maintenance, and repair of all of its tissues and organ systems.

Dr. Edward Howell, a pioneer in enzyme research has proven that a diet of cooked foods causes rapid, premature death in mice, and that the speed of premature death is directly connected to the temperature at which the food is cooked.

Dr. Howell's research also suggests that enzyme depleted foods rob your body of its enzyme potential and may reduce your life span. Digestion of enzyme depleted food is an extremely energy-consuming task for the body. This is why we often feel tired after a big meal.

> *The effects of cooked foods on the body include an increase in white blood cells or leukocytes. This increase is needed to transport enzymes to the digestive tract, however after eating raw food there is no substantial increase in leukocytes, showing that the body has to work much harder to produce and transport enzymes for digestion after a meal of cooked food.*
>
> *Leukocytosis increase is indicative of an acute illness or infection in the body. During acute dis-ease, enzyme levels rise. During chronic dis-ease the body enzyme levels are decreased. The pancreas and digestive tract are weakened, for example, during diabetes, cancer or chronic intestinal problems.*
> *-Influence of Food Cooking on the Blood Formula of Man*
>
> Dr. Paul Kautchakoff

Every bite of raw food provides your body with enzymes. Enzyme supplements taken with every meal will also add to your enzyme supply.

During my healing and even still today, I make it a habit to carry enzyme supplements in my purse for those times I find myself eating outside my home.

Enzyme supplements are an extract of energy food and designed to improve digestion. It is best to take an enzyme supplement to support your body in breaking down the foods you eat or you can use up what little bank of enzymes you have left. Digestive enzymes have been clinically proven to show, the more enzymes feed to the body, the quicker the body can repair, restore and strengthen itself.

### Probiotics

You may see on some of the commercial yogurts and other dairy products offer a mention of having
probiotics. Buyer beware! Dairy produces a lot of mucus in the body therefore lowering the immune system and causing more digestive issues. There is a balance to keep in mind when looking to get your probiotic intake from dairy.

Intestinal microbes can die off by the millions with illness, stress, medication use, and poor diet, but what we eat is the most important factor in keeping the gut healthy. Good bacteria feast on fiber. The "bad" guys love refined sugar, flour and animal products.

Greatly consider taking probiotics while you're taking antibiotics, and for at least two weeks afterwards. Antibiotics can be life-saving and absolutely essential – when used judiciously – but it's so important to support the good bacteria in growing and developing once the bad strains have been decimated.

Probiotics come in a wide range of formulations, from encapsulated beads to powders to entericcoated capsules. I typically go for the oral capsules and use the powdered ones as in implant when I am doing an enema or colon hydrotherapy.

A quality probiotic should combine several beneficial bacteria such as Saccharomyces, Lactobacillus Acidophilus and Bididobacteria in the billions.

### pH Balance: Acid / Alkaline

If we eat too many acid producing foods we become over acidic, and our immunity to disease is weakened. When the body holds onto waste, it produces an extremely acidic environment, also known as acidosis.

We should eat about 80% alkaline producing foods and 20% acid producing foods. In taking more alkaline foods help the body to heal and regain its balanced chemistry.

Nitrazine paper will show you your pH levels by applying saliva and/or urine to the paper. Always perform the test either before eating or at least an hour after eating. The paper will change color to indicate the acidity or alkalinity of your system. You can pick up nitrazine pH strips at Whole Foods market.

You would think that citrus fruits (oranges, lemons, grapefruits) would have an acid effect on the body, the citric acid they contain actually has an alkaline effect on the system, converting to carbon dioxide and water.

> *The term pH, means "potential hydrogen", represents a scale for the relative acidity or alkalinity of a solution. Acidity refers to the pH of 0.1 to 6.9, alkalinity is 7.1 to 14, and neutral pH is 7.0. The numbers refer to how many hydrogen atoms are present compared to an ideal or standard solution. Normally, blood is slightly alkaline, at 7.35 to 7.45. Urine pH can range from 4.8 to 7.5, although normal is closer t 7.0*
>
> *-Alternative Medicine Definition Guid to Cancer, Future Medicine Publishing, 1997 Dr. Paul Kautchakoff*

The following table shows a listing of acid forming foods and alkaline forming foods.

## Acid-Forming Foods

- Alcohol
- Animal products
- Asparagus
- Beans
- Brussel sprouts
- Candy
- Canned Fruits
- Catsup
- Chickpeas
- Cocoa
- Coffee
- Cornstarch
- Eggs
- Fish
- Flour products
- Legumes
- Lentils
- Meat (chicken / pork / beef)
- Milk
- Mustard
- Noodles
- Oatmeal
- Olives
- Pasta
- Pharmaceuticals
- Shellfish
- Smoked fish
- Sugar

## Alkaline Forming Foods

- Almonds
- Apricots
- Avocados
- Beets
- Buckwheat
- Carrots
- Corn
- Dates
- Fruits
- Grapefruits
- Grapes
- Green leafy veggies
- Lemons
- Maple syrup
- Melons
- Millet
- Molasses
- Oranges
- Potatoes
- Raisins
- Soybeans

# Chapter Eleven

## COLON HYDROTHERAY

I remember a few years ago, before I had any awareness of internal cleansing, one of my co-workers back in New York was telling me about her first experience and she just raved about how great she felt. I noticed that Carla had lost some weight. She had gone from a size 14-16 to a size 8-10 in only a couple of months. She contributed her weight loss and surge of energy to her new cleansing regimen and she was very excited that she did not have to get on high blood pressure medication.

I also remember one of my guy friends telling me about his experience with colon cleansing. I was so surprised that he was doing this. At the time, Tony was a very handsome man, about early 40s. A ladies man, he was always well manicured and all about his health and fitness. He said he did colonics because he noticed how great his skin looked and it made his stomach flat, really defining his abs. But even more important, Tony mentioned that he was sleeping a lot better at night, his back didn't bother him anymore and his could maintain an erection all night long – this was the true prize!

Even after hearing these reviews about cleansing, it still took me a couple of more years before I stepped up to the plate to try it for myself. Man, if only I had started two years ago,

I probably never would have gotten myself into this fix. Then too, I probably would not have written this book either. Hmmm, do you see the gift?

So what is colon hydrotherapy? Colon hydrotherapy is a process of slowly irrigating the large intestinal system with warm purified water via the rectum. The process is not at all painful and actually the therapy can be very relaxing. The procedure is odorless and very sanitary. If you are going to a cleansing clinic your therapist should provide you with a covering before the procedure to maintain your dignity.

I have also discovered various home / portable cleansing units that provide the same therapeutic benefits as the units in the clinics. These units are light weight, compact and very user friendly and they do not require you to have any kind of certification. Best of all, you are in the privacy of your own home.

If you are considering purchasing a private unit and have never had a colon hydrotherapy treatment before, it is my strong suggestion that you visit a certified colon hydrotherapist, at least for your first session. You can find one online at www.i-act.org.

Colon Hydrotherapy only takes about 30-45 minutes per session and you can continue with your day as usual. The experience is different for everyone. Some people feel a sense of clarity, like a fog has been lifted. Some people feel super charged with energy while some may feel very tired initially after their session. The reason for the lethargy after a treatment is likely due to the fact that your body really took on an internal aerobic session to release all of the old waste.

There are two different methods for colon hydrotherapy typically used in most cleansing clinics. One is called an open unit, the other is called a closed unit. I personally like both, but if I had to choose, I would probably go with the closed unit.

### Open Unit Colon Hydrotherapy

Open unit colon hydrotherapy is very effective and contrary to what may be believed, open unit cleansing is very clean and odorless too. This particular unit does give the client an opportunity to be in solitude while their body is processing the waste, however, it does not help the client to understand how their body is processing if the therapist is not there in the room to open up that dialog.

It has been my experience that a lot of (open unit) colonic technicians of leave the clients in the room during the entire session of the therapy without ever checking on them. This I find unacceptable, but this is just my personal and professional opinion.

### Closed Unit Colon Hydrotherapy

This system requires a trained colon hydrotherapist to be with the client during the entire procedure. Your therapist is there to monitor the water pressure and the waste product as it passes through the viewing tube. By opening up dialog with the client, the therapist is able to offer more information as to how your body is processing the removal of the waste and what supplements might support better digestion.

Waste is evacuated through a medical grade plastic tubing attached to the colon hydrotherapy instrument, and eliminated via a drainage line. This method is odorless and exceptionally sanitary.

### My First Experiences with Colonics

Now I have to tell you when I really got started with my first series of colon hydrotherapy treatments during my wellness rehabilitation I was not prepared for what I was about to discover about my body.

So, here it was, I was only taking in liquid nutrition – no solid foods at all. I was day four into my cleanse and during my first colon hydrotherapy treatment my body flushed a lot of waste. Things really did not get interesting until the second week of my cleanse and I was on my forth colon hydrotherapy treatment. Now remember, I'm not eating any solid foods at all; however my body was releasing waste like I had been eating a herd of elephants! Where in the world was all this stuff coming from? This was a huge paradigm shift for me.

## Age Old Mucus

As I continued on my cleanse, with each colon hydrotherapy treatment I was expecting to get to a point where there would be nothing to release, just water flushing though. Well that never happened. Every time I went in for my treatment, my body was processing out waste. There was so much mucus in my system that it looked like I was releasing thin sheets of skin. It was mucus that had accumulated in my body over the years from my dead food diet and constipation.

When I got to my last colonic treatment of this first series, number 20 to be exact, it was the last day of my first fast (Did you get all that?). Like any other treatment all was going well and then something totally different began to happen about half way through my session. I began sweating, my eyes were tearing and I had chills like it was below zero degrees. Then came this slight feel of nausea. This went on for about ten minutes before my body passed something that slowly oozed through the colonic view tube like black sludge. The sight of what was in the view tube startled me. *"What is that?"* I asked my therapist, *"This is likely what is making you sick, and we have just scratched the surface."* Was her reply as she googled the tube in utter fascination.

I always felt great after my colonic therapy sessions. Heck, I would usually leave my session and go right back to my daily tasks at hand, but this time I felt something remarkably different. For one thing, I was drained and all I wanted to do was go home and lay down.

Although I was very tired, my body felt lighter – lighter than how I usually felt after a colonic session. It was more like empty. When I went outside, the daylight was almost blinding and painful for my eyes to take on. The dull ache I did not know I was experiencing was no longer there. I once read something in one of my wellness books that stated some people never know how sick they are until they experience health.

Instead of my usual romping around after my session, I went home and laid down to rest. Because I had done so much reading and research, I was not too concerned about how weak I was feeling. I understood that my body just endured an inner battle to rid itself of the plastered waste it had been holding onto for years. I went home, and slept for about twelve hours straight.

When I woke up the next morning at about 4:30, I had another bowel release of that black sludge with sheets of mucus. My experience on the commode at home was not as dramatic as my experience at the colonic center, thank goodness. What I experienced next was simply remarkable.

When I looked in the mirror, my skin had a very bright glow to it and the whites of my eyes were actually white – not grey or yellow or bloodshot – but white! For the first time in a long time, my lower back was not bothering me and my joints felt very limber.

Prior to all of this cleansing, my vision was beginning to blur and I found myself needing to wear reading glasses. The reason why the light was so painful was that for the first time in a long time, I was able to see. This sentence alone takes on many meanings, far beyond the physical.

That last session of my first series of colonics turned a huge corner in the progress of my healing. My healing was turning into something far more than a physical transformation, it was an awakening. Something in me knew that I had a connection with God / the Universe that did not need a middleman to interpret my meditation (listening for God) or my prayers (speaking with God).

That morning during my quiet time, just as clear as a bell, God did speak to me. *"Your ministry is in your healing."*

### Colon Hydrotheapist vs. Colonic Technician

There is a difference between a colon hydrotherapist and a colonic technician, although if you were to ask, you would likely hear that there is no difference. Trust me on this – there is a difference, although they are both (rather they should be) professionally educated, trained and certified. Be sure to check on www.i-act.org (International Association for Colon Hydrotherapy).

A colonic therapist is a trained professional that coaches his/her clients through their cleansing and wellness process, engaging in dialog to help the client understand how they can better their health through internal cleansing, diet and supplementation. Because the therapist is with the client during the entire session observing the matter as it passes out of the body, the therapist can share theories as to why the client may be experiencing digestive challenges.

A colonic technician sets the clients up in the room, turns on the water and leaves the room. When clients time is up the technician enters the room, turns off the water and then cleans the unit after each session. Very little interaction or dialog is exchanged. Now, there are a few therapists that actually stay with their clients during an open session cleanse, or at the very least, check on them periodically. This select handful of therapist actually coach the clients through the cleansing process, but there is a greater majority that do not. The ones that do not are what I refer to as colonic technicians.

Colon hydrotherapy is a very intimate treatment and it is my opinion that it should be regarded as such. When a client comes into a wellness center for cleansing, they are not just there to wash and run. I believe it is the therapist's job to share their understanding with the client on what can be done to support their cleansing and wellness goals and not just lock them in a room with some running water and then collect a payment afterward.

Now there are alternatives to therapist or technician assisted colon hydrotherapy, one would be an enema and the other would be to purchase your own personal colonic unit.

### Colonic Treatments at Home

There are some wonderful and inexpensive portable / home colonic units that offer the same deep cleansing and release as the stationary clinical units. Also, with these units, you do not need certification or a prescription to purchase them. If you log onto www.madisoncarlista.com, you will find information about these wonderful units.

Remember what I shared earlier in the book about alkaline water? Well one of the most tremendous benefits of having a home colonic unit is that you can use the alkaline water in your cleansing. This has such tremendous effects for the colon. There are some wonderful educational (although visually squalid) videos on YouTube by Dr. Hiromi Shinya, MD. He provides several gastrointestinal endocosopy assessments of clients that have cleansed with alkaline water.

Some of the patients suffered from years of elimination issues, colon issues and even pre-cancerous conditions. The before and after impressions are nothing short of miraculous, and most in relatively short periods of time. Log onto the web and type in the following address to be taken directly to the YouTube video:

http://www.youtube.com/watch?v=han3AfjevOc

Word of caution, the videos are very vivid examination of his client's large intestinal organs before, with all of the hardened mucus lining, waste and some parasites. But honest to goodness, the view of the same patient afterward is, like I said, nothing short of amazing!

In the video, Dr. Shinya is promoting the Kangen Water System. Since it has come to America, of course it is a multi-level marketing business and the water system is almost $5,000. Although the system is wonderful, it is a bit overpriced, in order to pay the distributors. I have found a water system that is just as tremendous a quality as Kangen at more than half the price. You can log onto www.madisoncarlista.com to find the alkaline water system and get an additional 10% off the cost.

Again, I strongly suggest having your first colonic experience with a professionally trained and certified colon hydrotherapist.

The internal cleansing industry has been meeting some challenge here and there. For instance, in Texas, you **must** have a prescription from a medical doctor. The catch 22 is that most doctors won't give a prescription for colonic therapy. Now this is a whole 'nother subject matter. A lot of this has to do with politics and a lot has to do with ignorance. Did you know that the typical medical student only gets an average of 5-10 hours of nutritional / dietary education? Guess how much information they get on cleansing? None, nada, zilch, zero, nothing! If a patient has a bowel impaction, they would rather put on a rubber glove and dig the impaction out of the rectum. Now I know this sounds gross, but this what conventional medicine believes to be the best method of hardened fecal removal.

I don't know about you, but it has been my experience from childhood that when I had to wash dishes after my grandmother cooked lasagna, I would have to soak the glass Pyrex dish because the noodles, sauce and cheese had hardened. After a good water soaking, guess what? I could practically rinse the dish clean. Hmmm, is it possible the same could be done inside the colon? Again, duh!

Most doctors are quick to tell their patient that colon hydrotherapy could rupture the colon or clean all of the "good" bacteria out of the colon.

To this I say, study and show yourself approved. If your body is riddled with yeast and parasites and your bowels are not moving. Trust me, you don't have to worry about washing out the good bacteria. There is none to wash out! But again, do your homework

**Enema**

With colon hydrotherapy, the water has the opportunity to negotiate throughout the entire large intestinal system; an enema only cleanses the lower part of the bowel. With an enema you are missing about four feet of colon. Fleece enemas use high-volume pressurized fills, sometimes fatiguing the colon.

When it comes to taking an enema, I prefer to use the old fashioned red hot water bottle enema / douche bag (you can go onto www.madisoncarlista.com to order one or you can pick one up at your nearest pharmacy). Remember the kind grandma use to keep hanging in the bathroom? Yep, that's exactly what I'm talking about. I personally keep two enema bags. One stays in my suitcase (I NEVER travel without it), and the other I keep at home for a quick pick me up (yeah, seriously).

You can do an enema while sitting on the toilet in a squatted position, or even better, position yourself in the bathtub – lay down and let the water flow into your colon. Try to hold it for as long as you can before you get up to release in the commode.

Listen, some water to cleanse is better than no water at all and here again is the best opportunity to use alkaline water for your cleansing.

Whether you do an open session colonic, a closed session colonic or enema, just give yourself the gift of cleansing so your body can release.

You bath the outside of your body every day, right? Why wouldn't you bath the inside as well? The inside of your body is experiencing more filth and grime and for longer periods of time than the outside. Something to think about.

**Toilet Etiquette**

The modern day toilet is the one of the major health disparities relative to digestion, colon and pelvic dis-eases.

Here again, I have something that I must share with you. This is a bit of historical background on the toilet:

*Man, like his fellow primates, has always used the squatting position for elimination. Infants of every culture instinctively adopt this posture to relieve themselves. Although it may seem strange to someone who has spent his entire life deprived of the experience, this is the way the human body was designed to function.*

*And this is the way our ancestors performed their bodily functions until the middle of the 19th century. Before that time, chair-like toilets had only been used by royalty and the disabled. But with the advent of indoor plumbing in the 1800's, the throne-like water closet was invented to give ordinary people the same "dignity" previously reserved for kings and queens. The plumber and cabinet maker who designed it had no knowledge of human physiology – and sincerely believed that they were improving people's lives.*

*The new device symbolized the "progress" and "creativity" of western civilization. It showed that Man could "improve" on Nature and transcend the primitive cultural practices followed by the poor "benighted" natives in the colonies. The "White Man's Burden" typified the condescending Victorian attitude toward other races and cultures.*

*The British plumbing industry moved quickly to install indoor plumbing and water closets throughout the country. The great benefits of improved sanitation caused people to overlook a major ergonomic blunder: The sitting position makes elimination difficult and incomplete, and forces one to strain.*

*Those who could not overlook this drawback had to keep silent, because the subject was considered unmentionable. Furthermore, how could they criticize the "necessary" used by Queen Victoria herself? (Hers was gold-plated, befitting the self-styled "Empress of India.")*

*So, like the Emperor's New Clothes, the water closet was tacitly accepted. It was a grudging acceptance, as evidenced by the popularity of "squatting stools" sold in the famous department store, Harrods of London. As shown below on the left, these footstools merely elevated one's feet in a crude attempt to imitate squatting.*

*The rest of Western Europe, as well as Australia and North America, did not want to appear less civilized than Great Britain, whose vast empire at the time made it the most powerful country on Earth. So, within a few decades, most of the industrialized world had adopted "The Emperor's New Throne."*

*150 years ago, no one could have predicted how this change would affect the health of the population. But today, many physicians blame the modern toilet for the high incidence of a number of serious ailments. Westernized countries have much higher rates of colon and pelvic disease.*

Seven advantages of Squatting:

1. Makes elimination faster, easier and more complete. This helps prevent "fecal stagnation", a prime factor in colon cancer, appendicitis and IBS.

2. Protects the nerves that control the prostate, bladder and uterus from becoming stretched and damaged.

3. Securely seals the ileocecal valve, between the colon and the small intestine. In the conventional sitting position, this valve is unsupported and often leaks during evacuation, contaminating the small intestine.

4. Relaxes the puborectalis muscle which normally chokes the rectum in order to maintain continence.

5. Uses the thighs to support the colon and prevent straining. Chronic straining on the toilet can cause hernia, diverticulosis, and pelvic organ prolapsed.

6. A highly effective, non-invasive treatment for hemorrhoids, as shown by published clinical research.

7. For pregnant women, squatting avoids pressure on the uterus when using the toilet. Daily squatting helps prepare the mother-to-be for a more natural delivery.

## Won't I Wash Away All My Good Stuff?

There is a huge myth about colon hydrotherapy washing away all of the good bacteria. Well, here's something to consider – maybe you should not bathe everyday as you may wash all of the oils out of your skin. Sounds crazy, right? The same with colon hydrotherapy. First of all, if your bowels are not eliminating after each and every meal, you very likely do not have a lot of good bacteria to work with. If you have not done any kind of cleansing at all or only minimal cleansing of your bowels, just assume that you do not have to worry about washing away all of your good bacteria.

The body naturally produces yeast, but when yeast becomes over populated in the system it can wreak havoc on the immune system. This is referred to as candidiasis. Yeast is a breeding ground for all other forms of parasitic infections, compromising the immune system.

Something else to consider is the use of antibiotics. Let's take the word antibiotic and break it down:

**Anti** – Against          **Biotic** - Life

Antibiotics are designed to kill off the harmful living bacteria, but it also kills off the beneficial living bacteria as well. It's no wonder after a series of antibiotic intake, women end up with crazy yeast infections.

Yeast, also recognized as candidiasis should not be taken lightly. Research suggests that candidiasis may be connected with immune disorders such as AIDS, cancer and other life-threatening illnesses.

> *The prevalence of bowel dis-eases (hemorrhoids, appendicitis, polyps, ulcerative colitis, IBS and colon cancer) are similar in South African whites and in populations of prosperous western countries. Among rural South African Blacks with a traditional lifestyle, these dis-eases are very uncommon or almost unknown.*
> *-Israel Journal of Medical Science*

I can remember during one of my physical exams a few years ago I asked my doctor if it would be a good idea for me to start taking acidophilus since I had been on and off antibiotics throughout the year for colds and flu. My licensed, Manhattan NY, $350 office visit MD looked at me with eyes glazed over and asked, *"What is acidophilus?"* Before I could answer she quickly interjected, *"I've never heard of such thing. It's probably just some old wives tale."* I knew then I was on my own to figure out the truth, because clearly this lab coat space cadet was not the one.

I have a theory about yeast or candidiasis. Yeast is a bacterial parasite. It is my belief that yeast breads and sets the breeding ground for other parasitic infections. Remember, like attracts like. Cancer, diabetes, AIDS and every other dis-ease is nothing more than a parasitic infection. I believe and it has been my personal experience that if you work to rid the body of excess yeast and get the pH balance of the body to balance the body has a greater chance of overcoming health challenges. Things that make you go, hmmmm.

My experience has been that the body can balance itself with the support of an organic diet with living foods, alkaline water, nutritional supplementation, cleansing and probiotics.

### Autointoxication

Trust me when I tell you that it is better to be pro-active than re-active. There are many conditions that respond to colon hydrotherapy. Colon hydrotherapy can help reverse autointoxication. When your body is ill and riddled with dis-ease, you are suffering from autointoxication.

Dr. John H. Tilden, MD is a renowned natural healer and author. He made a powerful statement regarding his interpretation of autointoxication which he refers to as toxemia.

116

> *Autointoxication is the process whereby the body literally poisons itself by maintaining a cesspool of decaying matter in its colon. This inner cesspool can contain as high a concentration of harmful bacteria as a cesspool under a house. The toxins released by the decay process get into the bloodstream and travel to all parts of the body. Every cell in the body is affected, and many forms of sickness can result. Because it weakens the entire system, autointoxication can be a causative factor for nearly any dis-ease.*
>
> *-The Colon Health Handbook, Rockridge Publishing Co.*

Without toxemia there can be no dis-ease. All dis-eases are the same fundamentally. The cause travels back to toxemia, caused by enervation (lack of nerve energy), which checks elimination and induces a toxic state. Every chronic dis-ease starts with toxemia and a toxic crisis.

When the nervous system is normal – when there is nerve energy – man is normal and immune to dis-ease. Dis-ease begins to manifest only when environments and personal habits use up energy faster than it is renewed.

Dr. Bernard Jensen, DC, another world renowned natural healer summarizes the results of his experience:

*"In the 50 years I've spent helping people to overcome disability and disease, it has become crystal clear that poor bowel management lives at the root of most people's health problems. In treating over 500,000 patients, it is the bowel that invariably has to be cared for before effective healing can take place. Trying to take care of any symptom in the body without good elimination is futile."*

It is better to be proactive about your health and healing than to wait to the point that you have to make a change or else. Some of the common symptoms of autointoxication or toxicity overload can be easily eliminated by cleansing and simple lifestyle adjustments.

- Constipation
- Depression
- Fatigue
- Frequent Colds
- Halitosis (bad breath)
- Indigestion
- Obesity

- Headaches
- Acne
- Skin Rashes
- Sinus Congestion
- Joint Stiffness / Aches
- Menstrual Challenges
- Allergies

## Cancer and Autointoxication

> *Women who have 2 or fewer bowel movements per week have 4 times the risk of breast and reproductive dis-ease as women who have 1 or more bowel movements per day.*
>
> *The same statistic appeals to men as well. Men who have 4 or fewer bowel movements per week have 8 times the risk of prostate dis-ease.*
>
> *-Saturday Evening Post*

*Alright Madison, I see you are quite radical about this whole colon cleansing thing.*

OK, I suppose from the outside looking in I may come across as a radical, but I just know what cleansing has done for me. But, I will also tell you that it would be ignorant and irreverent to claim that colon hydrotherapy alone, even with the alkaline water reversed my cancer.

I employed a diversity of regimes during my healing rehabilitation and I still utilize these same practices as my anti-aging and wellness protocols. As you read further in the book you will gain more insight to the methods of my madness and hopefully recognize the silver lining of sanity.

Constipation can cause you to be poisoned by your own waste, a state known as autointoxication. Even short-term constipation is not good.

Indigestion, gas, bloating, allergies and hay fever, arthritis, and even colon cancer could be considered huge red flag signs of autointoxication caused by constipation.

Your health and energy depend on your body moving out waste. Bowel movements should ideally occur for every meal you intake throughout the day. If you consume three meals a day, you should eliminate three times a day. Anything less may leave toxic waste in the body.

When the toxicity level in the colon rises, these poisons can back-up into the bloodstream and into the liver. This means that the liver must handle them a second time and this leads to liver overload. When the liver is overloaded it can't handle the new toxins coming in because it has too much to do. These toxics further back up into the blood stream.

The increased blood levels of impurities and toxic spillage goes from the blood into other organs like the brain, heart, skin and kidneys. At this point systemic symptoms can really become significant such as: generalized fatigue, bad breath, foul body odor, depression, poor sleep, and moodiness.

Essentially, each of our cells now gets back the waste that they have already dumped. This is autointoxication. If you have low energy, brain fog, arthritis, autoimmune dis-ease, high blood pressure and even diabetes, this may be the underlying cause.

**Parasites: The Nucleus of Cancer**

One of my favorite authors, Hulda R. Clark, PhD, ND believes that all cancers are from solvents, contaminates and parasites. Solvents can be acquired through your skin and your breathing. Dr. Clark maintains that contaminants are contributing factors to cancer, but holds parasites as the main culprits. The solvents that are acquired through the breath and skin contact go into the bloodstream and provide an additional stream of nourishment to various parasitic bacteria. Dr. Clark believed and taught that each cancer is associated with a certain type of parasite. Remember what I said about yeast? Yeast is a breeding ground for other parasites.

# IONIC CLEANSE

I love Ionic Cleanse foot baths. This is another very simple yet exceptional therapy. Your feet are set in a tub of warm sea salt water with an electrical unit that produces negative and positive ions in the body. Those ions attach to bacteria and are dawn out through the soles of your feet. The pores on the bottom on your feet are the largest pores of the body.

It is amazing to watch the water change from clear to yellow, orange, brown and even black with foam. This is all indicative of the body pulling waste from various organs throughout the body.

If you were to actually take a sample of the water from the residue of your ion cleanse and put it under a microscope you would be able to see the living bacteria pulled from your cells.

I have found the ionic cleansing is excellent for ridding my body of heavy metals and yeast. It has also been my experience that ion cleansing has helped with joint and muscle discomfort too.

### Oh Yeah, a Word about Yeast

There is a huge misconception that only women get yeast infections. Well, today is the dawn of a new understanding, because guess what? Men are just as prone to yeast infections as women are and men can pass a yeast infection to a woman. Yep – yeast or candida is an opportunitistic fungus that normally inhabits the mouth, throat, gastrointestinal tract and for women, the vagina. By the time women realize it vaginally, it has pretty much spread throughout the body.

The signs for yeast infection with men will manifest itself as jock itch, athlete's foot or some other skin affliction. Yeast may even manifest itself as a discharge from the penis, but typically the man does not get the same kind of signs as the woman. And yes, a yeast infection is still transferable from woman to man and from man to woman.

Remember, yeast starts in the digestive tract. With that being said it is easily understood that if you were to change the environment of the gut then likely the symptoms will change as well. How would you change the environment? Through your diet! It has been my experience from reading and personal experimentation that yeast feeds off of flour, sugars, animal products and processed foods, long term use of antibiotics, birth control pills, painkillers, regular use of cortisone-type drugs, stimulants and depressants, diabetes, and various viral dis-eases.

# HYPERBARIC CHAMBER

Hyperbaric Oxygen Therapy (HBOT) is definitely one of my secret weapons for anti-aging, but it was during my healing transformation that this treatment laid the foundation for my overall well-being.

Oxygen deficiency is often overlooked and yet it is vital for health as it is the single most vital element your body needs. At the cellular level, oxygen is required for proper function. Not only does oxygen fuel the body, it supports the immune system by destroying toxic substances. Anaerobic bacteria, fungi and viruses (hmmm, would this mean HPV, HIV, and any other type of V(irus?) have a common intolerance for oxygen; they cannot survive in an oxygen rich environment.

Your body's vital functions are enhanced by increased availability of oxygen. Oxygen is our primary source of energy. Increased pressure in addition stimulates blood flow and decreases inflammation.

Oxygen therapy has a tremendously calming effect and enhances sleep. This treatment also supports absorption of nutrients and improved digestion.

During HBOT you are placed in a specially designed chamber, the pressure in the chamber is increased, and 100% oxygen is breathed.

Alveolar oxygen pressure is increased, causing a rise in blood oxygen content, resulting in enhanced tissue oxygen delivery. The amount of pressure increase and the length of time are determined by the condition being treated. Oxygen therapy is usually between 1 to 2 hours at full pressure.

There are HBOT clinics you can go to or you can purchase your own personal chamber. Go to www.madisoncarlista.com and there you will find one of what I believe to be the best on the market for personal HBOT.

Most of the women I know spend their money on shoes, clothes and other depreciative trinkets. I'm the type of woman that would list a personal HBOT chamber as one of those guilty pleasures I would invest to have in my home.

### A Word about Deep Breathing

I understand that not everyone can afford a hyperbaric chamber or maybe they do not have access to a chamber in their town. The next best thing to HBOT is plain ol' deep breathing.

Have you ever noticed a baby while she / he is sleeping? What about a cat or dog? If you pay attention, you will see that they breathe deeply, from their diaphragm. As we age and take on the daily stresses of life, we have a tendency to hold our breath, in anticipation, anxiety, repressed anger, you get the picture. Well during all of this "holding on"(and a lot of this is purely emotional) we have subconsciously trained ourselves to all but stop breathing. Now we just breathe enough to keep us functioning, barely. Think I'm kidding? Take notice of your breath now. Where are you breathing from? If you are not consciously aware, you are probably breathing from your chest - little wimpy, shallow breaths causing oxygen deficiency. By using your diaphragm as well as your upper chest, you will be able to take in more oxygen enhancing your healthy cells while suppressing the growth of the unhealthy cells. Of course, the fresher the air the better. If you live in the city, take a journey to the park and sit amongst the trees or better yet, if you can get to the mountains – Go!

I love plants and try to keep as many as I can around my home. Plants add such a wonderful vibe to my home and the oxygen they provide is priceless. More than just decoration, plants are life preservers.

Another thing that helps me to focus on my breathing is meditation. Just sitting still and allowing all to just be. This also offers a great opportunity for me to just listen for God.

Last but surely not least is cardio or aerobic exercise. Exercise increases the capacity of both the heart and lungs, thus getting more oxygen to the cells.

## LYMPHATIC STIMULATION

The lymphatic system is the only structure in the body that does not have its own pumping mechanism. The only way the lymphatic system is stimulated is through compression, massage therapy or exercise.

The greatest mistake made in conventional medicine is that if the patient has a tumor, massage is eliminated. It has been my personal experience that massage is one of the best ways to drain the lymphatics. My mentor Versandra Kennebrew can really go on and on about this subject alone. Not only is massage beneficial for the purpose of physical stimulation, but the whole process of touch therapy is powerful!

Versandra has a worldwide organization called *Touch is Great*. She is a professional massage therapist and educator. This woman is powerful and her passion in sharing her understanding about the power of touch therapy is transformational. There is more to massage than just manipulating muscles. When done with pure intention, the therapy is truly healing. For more information about Versandra's educational ministry, log onto www.touchisgreat.com.

I recognize that physical touch may not be for everyone and there were many times during my healing transition that I did not feel like being touched because of my own emotional and sometimes physical sensitivity.

Another great stimulation for the lymphatic system is endermologie. I haven't found a home unit for this particular therapy, but I can tell you that aside from the lymphatic stimulation the esthetic benefits are so awesome!

Endermologie is provided by a spa specialist that uses a handheld unit that rolls and suctions the skin. The therapy is very relaxing and it is excellent for breaking up cellulite and giving dimpled skin a smoother firmer appeal.

**Compression Wear for Lymphatic Stimulation**

Another excellent stimulation for the lymphatic system and is very complementary for aftercare of endermology is wearing a compression garment. When compression is engineered to apply a balanced and accurate surface pressure over specific body parts, it triggers an acceleration of blood flow.

An orthopedically engineered gradient compression garment can enhance blood flow and venous return, increasing oxygen delivery to working muscles and more rapidly eliminating lactic acid and waste.

For the past few months I had been hearing about this garment called Body Magic. Someone came to me talking about wearing a girdle to drop 2-3 pounds in 10 minutes. This did not interest me, at all. What did get my attention was the fact that this garment was developed by an orthopaedic surgeon. My first thought was, *"What does a surgeon have to do with a piece of lingerie"*?

During my healing transformation, I was introduced to and wore a compression garment, long before the Body Magic craze. Not all compression garments are made alike. The garments I chose to wear were developed by an orthopaedic surgeon. They were quite functional, but not very attractive. Just your plain ol' medical beige no thrills, no frills super medical grade lycra wear.

Today I wear a Body Magic compression sport shirt which is great for my workouts and I also wear the Body Magic full compression garment that provides upper and lower back support, making my poster tall and erect, which also opens up my chest for better breathing. The structure of the full wear garment provides pelvic bridge support, buttock support and it helps with proper placement of the internal organs, lifting the large intestine and the pelvic, taking pressure off of the lower colon. The buttock panel also takes pressure off of the rectum. Overall, this provides is a huge support for the digestive and elimination system.

An added plus to wearing Body Magic is that it is actually a sexy piece of lingerie that slenderizes the body. Just the esteem from your clothes fitting better does wonders for the immune system! Trust me on this one.

## FIR SAUNA (Far InfraRed)

There are conventional saunas and then there is FIR sauna. Conventional saunas heat up the air in the room sometimes to a searing temperature capable of damaging respiratory and vision. Conventional saunas are not recommended for those with cardiac or diabetic conditions.

Sweating is good as it helps to stimulate the lymphatic glands and accelerates the body to detox waste through the skin. It has been my experience that when my health was at a greater challenge, FIR was a safer and much more comfortable alternative to conventional saunas.

FIR sauna therapy produces the same wave currency as the sun. FIR heat is a form of naturally occurring energy that heats objects by direct light conversion (DLC). DLC warms only the object (the body) and does not raise the temperature of the surrounding free air.

All life requires FIR heat from the sun. FIR heat is not ultraviolet radiation but a narrow band of energy within the 5.6 to 15 micron level. This type of energy travels 2-3" beneath the skin's surface to increase circulation and nourish damaged tissue.

It is typically in our fat cells where waste and toxicity will also lie dormant. Toxins such as sodium, alcohol, nicotine, cholesterol and carcinogenic heavy metals (cadmium, lead, zinc, nickel) and mercury accumulate in the body just in everyday life. The body can eliminate most of these toxins by sweating but the process can be sometimes slow. FIR stimulates the sweat glands that cleanse and detoxify the skin. FIR just speeds up the process.

I still use FIR Sauna therapy just for how it benefits my skin. FIR heat improves circulation, expels dirt and chemicals and removes dead cells on the surface of the skin. All of these benefits lead to a more soft yet firm completion.

# Chapter Twelve

## THE BUSINESS OF CANCER:
### A Jaded Love Story

The cancer industry is conservatively estimated to be worth an annual $75 to $100 billion, including treatment and research. If by chance some simple and inexpensive replacement for chemotherapy, radiation and drug treatment were announced by the media all US medical schools would be knocking on the doors of bankruptcy. Cancer treatments in the hospitals average $60,000 to $85,000 per person per cancer and that cost is rising. Cancer equals huge dollars.

Look at the numbers of people affected with cancer. Just three to four generations ago 33 people were diagnosed with cancer in their lifetime. Now, one in three people are diagnosed. There is more money thrown at the research for cancer with new drugs being introduced every time we turn around. The drugs are only treating the symptoms, but not the cancer itself.

The "war on cancer" is a losing battle for the patient. So my position on this war? Stop fighting the war and focus on winning the battle instead!

My observation is that we have a multi-billion dollar cancer control industry that mainly conducts damage control by treating the symptoms, not the basic underlying cause.

My research has shown me that there are plenty of known cures for cancer that the medical industry is aware of, but the money is not in the cure. The money is in the dis-ease itself.

In Paul Zane Pilzer's book, *The Next Trillion*, he mentions how decisions are made to keep America on a drug maintenance program for sickness and dis-ease. Let's say the pharmaceutical industry has been offered insight of a brand new drug that could totally cure cancer, diabetes, sickle cell, whatever you want to name the dis-ease. The drug costs them only pennies to manufacture and they could sell it to each patient for $150 a pill.

Now let's say the industry has been shown an alternative drug that helps to maintain the dis-ease, *not cure it, but maintain it*. This drug only costs pennies to manufacture as well, and as a "maintenance therapy" they can sell it to patients for $3.00 per pill per day for the rest of the patient's life. Now, put your business hat on. From a profit standpoint, what looks like the better deal to you?

I know I may come across as a radical against conventional medicine. This is not my intention at all. I am just very pro education about alternative theories in health and healing.

Like alternative wellness, conventional medicine has its place. If I should go out and break my leg skiing, don't take me to a massage therapist. Please, take me to a medical doctor so they can help to reset my bone. From there I will also incorporate what I understand about nutrition, supplementation and other therapies to help speed the recovery of the fracture as well.

Ideally, conventional medicine and alternative wellness should work hand in hand. There is already a name for this union, it is called CAM (Conventional Alternative Medicine). Unfortunately, there is a great deal of bureaucracy swirling around holistic wellness. The government is positioning itself to control natural foods and natural therapies. Why? Because according to a national statistic from 2005, Americans spent over $30 billion in alternative therapies – Out of Pocket. The government, pharmaceutical, food or any of the other bureaucratic agencies did not get any slice of this income.

## Cancer's Annual Treatment Cost (U.S)

| | | | |
|---|---|---|---|
| *Breast:* | $6.6 billion | *Uterine:* | $1.6 billion |
| *Cololorectal:* | $6.5 billion | *Melanoma:* | $1.1 billion |
| *Lung:* | $5 billion | *Leukemia:* | $1.1 billion |
| *Prostate:* | $4.7 billion | *Kidney:* | $1 billion |
| *Bladder:* | $2.2 billion | | |

Cervical / Ovarian / Stomach / Pancreatic: $610 million to $1 billion each.

*-An Alternative Medicine Definitive Guide to Cancer, 1997*

## More Accurate Testing for Cervical / Prostrate / and other Cancers

CSA is an awesome early detection test with close to 100% accuracy. This test offers a much more accurate answer at a fraction of the cost and inconvenience of the standard pap smear test.

*False negatives are common in pap smears, occurring in about 30% of all cases. The error rate for cervical cancer may be as high as 50%. A woman may have several false negative pap tests in a row before falling ill and finding out that she has actually developed cervical cancer. We are at the mercy of conventional cancer screening which detects cancer in its later stages of development.*

*-Acta Cytologica Medical Journal*
*-Diamond, et al, 1997*

The male version of the CSA test is the PSA test. Once again this provides a much more accurate rate of result than the standard, "okay, now turn your head and cough."

Another awesome test that I just read about covers the entire gamut of cancers. It is the AMAS Blood Test. This test is noted to detect any and all kinds of cancers up to 19 months before conventional medical tests can determine a lump or mass is present.

You will find information on how to get these tests in the Reference Guide in section three.

Be informed. If you or your loved one is facing cancer, of any kind, become an information hound. Do not just give your power over to the doctors and have them to "fix it". You fix it! Because of your lifestyle choices you were the one that got yourself into this situation, now take responsibility to get yourself out of it.

I'm not suggesting that you totally ignore what your doctor is telling you. I would be so out of place to do that, but what I am saying is make your doctor earn your money. Do your research, bring your findings to your doctor and compare notes. When it comes to natural or alternative medicine most doctors are very ignorant to anything outside of their conventional study of medicine. Doctors are educated to be post-active, not pro-active. Arm yourself with knowledge so that you can speak from a position of power and not from fear and panic.

**The JibJab Truth:**
**HPV ≠ Cervical Cancer?**

There is a huge push for young girls, starting at age 12 to get the Gardasil or Cervarix shot for cervical cancer. According to the CDC, the Human PapillomaVirus (HPV) is responsible for the surge in cervical cancer. What is their answer to this? Well a vaccination of course! Now what if I were to tell you that in 2003 the FDA knew, conclusively, that HPV does not cause cervical cancer at all?

Mike Adams, the Health Ranger brought up an interesting article on one of his video blogs. The FDA in 2003 issued a press release stating that most women who become infected with the HPV are able to eradicate the virus and suffer no apparent long term consequences to their health. In other words, the body's innate ability to seize the virus can do so on its own, without a vaccination, pill, poke, jab, etc.

If you haven't checked out Mike Adams, hurry to your internet and log onto www.healthranger.com. This man is full of wisdom in the field of alternative theories in health and healing. Absolutely one of my favorites!

I met and befriended a really awesome lady from Australia by the name of Angela Perin. Angela is absolutely fanatical about health and wellness. She and her husband Dennis live a totally holistic lifestyle, even down to home birthing their 3 daughters.

Angela has taken on a personal crusade to educate women about the cervical cancer vaccination, and remains a firm advocate of informed choice and revealing the truth. Following is an article she wrote titled, Fact or Fear, Cervical Cancer and the HPV Vaccine.

*Unless you've been living in isolation for the past couple of years, you would have found it almost impossible to avoid hearing about the risk of cervical cancer, and the two new HPV (Human Papillomavirus) vaccines (Gardasil and Cervarix) that have now been introduced as a prevention strategy against this disease.*

*In a revolutionary age where media campaigning has tremendous power and potential to infiltrate thinking and ideas on national and global scales, distinguishing fact from emotion becomes a confronting, yet subtle dilemma.*

*The platform for the introduction of these 2 new HPV vaccines onto the worldwide market has been on the basis of the threat and risk of cervical cancer, and has presented the same dilemma to potential recipients of these vaccines.*

*The problem is, although facts are a far more logical basis on which to make such a decision, emotion is often a far more powerful motivator for action or compliance in situations where health is the prime factor. And in this situation, the fear of cervical cancer has formed a very solid basis for the HPV vaccine campaigns.*

*There's certainly no question that cervical cancer disease can and does have serious (sometimes fatal) outcomes. However, equally so, any medical procedure, artificial drug, pharmaceutical product or vaccine by its very nature also carries with it varying degrees of risk - both temporary and permanent. This includes the HPV vaccines.*

*The unfortunate truth is that the bulk of media campaigning and information disseminated to the public has avoided, disguised or cleverly side-stepped pointing out the facts and health risks associated with the actual vaccines, which to date have included (but are not limited to): loss of consciousness, paralysis, Guillain Barre Syndrome, hospitalization, permanent disability and death.*

*The questions any female or parent (of daughters) considering this vaccine needs to ask themselves are these:*

- *Is cervical cancer as widespread and as serious a health risk as portrayed in media campaigns and by our health authorities?*
- *Is it merely coincidence that solid media campaigns against cervical cancer disease have been hand-in-hand with the introduction of these vaccines?*
- *Have all the facts regarding all the risks of both the disease and the vaccine been accurately revealed?*

*The challenge for any potential recipient is in identifying the true facts about the risk of cervical cancer versus the associated risks and benefits of the vaccine. Unfortunately, many recipients of these vaccines have based their decision on limited information provided in media campaigning that has ignored all the facts - resulting in decisions made on emotion rather than sound logical judgment.*

*Tragically in many cases, the associated health risks of the vaccine have resulted in more devastating and irreversible outcomes than an actual cervical cancer diagnosis. As challenging as it might be, you owe it to yourself to research the facts before deciding whether or not these vaccines are of benefit, and whether these benefits outweigh any potential risks.*

*By basing your decision on fact, not fear, your decision will be an informed one, and the one that's right for you in your individual situation. Whatever you decide, make it an informed one.*

The whole topic around the cervical cancer vaccines would be an entire other book. There is so much research and information that you need to consider. With that being said, you can go to my website www.madisoncarlista.com and download the exclusive expose': *Cervical Cancer Vaccine – The Truth: The Facts Every Female Must Know and Why!*

Well dear heart, you have been armed with the truth. Well, at least my perception of it anyway. What you do with it is up to you. Remember, sickness, dis-ease and aging starts from the inside out, not the outside in. If you want to restore your body, cease the aging process, heal your life – TAKE RESPONSIBILITY! All you need is innately within you.

*The illumination of the dark fact that most of what you have heard over your lifetime about cancer treatments is not the truth. At the very least, you have received an incomplete picture. If you believe the propaganda you have been fed and you develop cancer, it can cost you your life.*
*-An Alternative Medicine Definitive Guide to Cancer.*

# A FINAL THOUGHT

I want to make it a point to live my mission statement. It is my desire to do God's will and share my understanding of ultimate health and healing. I was fortunate in that I was able to recognize my teachers and mentors as they presented themselves to me, each one after the other.

Much of what I studied in the bible as I was growing up is making more sense to me now. My ongoing search for deeper understanding reveals so much that is taken out of context. As I cross reference my bible study with other ancient text like the Holy Koran, The Tibetan Book of the Dead, The Emerald Tablets and so forth, my understanding is anewed daily.

*My people are destroyed for lack of knowledge.*
Hosea 4:6

I know a lot of highly educated folks out here in this world and yet many of them are about to keel over dead for not understanding that their lack of knowledge is robbing them of their peace, their passion, their health, their happiness and their financial prosperity. Education and Knowledge are two totally different understandings.

*Study to show yourself approved.*
II Timothy 2:15

When God said study, (s)he was not just speaking of the King James Version of the Bible. Remember, history is always told by the concurer. Read, study and cross reference. One thing that I say to whatever group I may be speaking to is to not believe a word I say, as I can only come from my own understanding and experience. But when you have your own understanding and experience, the information has a whole new paradigm of interpretation.

I can't tell you how often people come up to me and ask what I did to overcome the diagnosis of advanced cervical cancer and how did I do it. What they are looking for is a quick step by step shortcut to glory. They are looking for a magic bullet. Here's a hint: THERE IS NO MAGIC BULLET!!!!

What I went through was not a walk in the park, nor was it an overnight sensation. I had to work to achieve it and I still have to work even that much more diligently to maintain it. But this holds true for anything in life.

Much of what I employed during my health transformation has become a staple in my lifestyle. I still cleanse, I still maintain a vegetarian / vegan diet, I still take my supplements and nutriceuticals, I still fast and I exercise my body regularly. I have become a certifiable gym rat!

Getting older and aging is not the same thing.
- Getting older relates to the passage of time.
- Aging relates to the breakdown of tissues in the body.
- The outward signs of aging include wrinkles, sagging, and gray hair.
- Getting older by itself does not cause aging.

Because of my lifestyle, I have the constitution of a woman more than half my age. My body is svelte and lean; my skin glows and I have an energetic attraction that pulls people into my aura. I attract the whos and whats that are calibrating at my same frequency or higher.

Energy begets energy. This transformation has set off a chain reaction. My income has doubled... tripled...and exploded exponentially! I went from looking swell but broke as hell to living well with the lifestyle to tell. My family relationships thrive and even my social circle of friends are different.

Since overcoming the diagnosis and prognosis, I have not looked back. When I find my energy waning or my skin begins to lose a bit of its luster, or if I am feeling on edge, I review my habits. I can always see where I have slipped up, so I just get back on track. Everything in relation to my life is about progression onward and ever upward. My intention is to share my knowledge with anyone and everyone that is in the space to listen and understand.

This is just the beginning of my ministry. This book launches the platform for $S^2O$ Spa Institute for Anti-Aging and Holistic Healing. I pray to remain obedient to spirit and attract the leadership to assure the facility lives up to the calling of its purpose. Right now, you can visit $S^2O$ Spa virtually through my website, www.madisoncarlista.com. There you will find a lot of the nutriceuticals and other products I have mentioned here in the book.

I am in a space of always growing. I never want to *know* anything, but just come to a new *understanding* of everything.

With this book and my message I will tour and speak, where ever God wants me to go, sharing more intimate details of my journey and my new understandings. I look forward to being with you again at some point in time.

Until then, I bid you ageless health, joy overflowing, financial prosperity and love.

I AM Madison Carlista and I am an infinite spiritual being and cervical cancer survivor.

# INDEX III

*All of the information provided in this section is
expounded upon on
www.madisoncarlista.com*

| | |
|---|---|
| AMAS Testing<br>Oncolab<br>36 The Fenway<br>Boston, MA 02215<br>800-922-8378<br>617-536-0850<br>www.oncolabinc.com | AMAS (Anti-Malignin Antibody Screen). Early cancer detection test with a documents 99% accuracy rating. |
| Onconix, Inc.<br>3455 University Parkway<br>Winston-Salem, NC 27106<br>www.onconix.net<br>336-408-3337<br>onconix.net/Index.htm | CSA Test (Cervical Cancer Blood Test). Highly accurate blood test identifies specific stages of dis-ease. Overcomes deficiencies of Pap smear. |
| PSA<br><br><br>www.directlabs.com/ | PSA Test (Prostate-specific Antigen) Highly accurate analysis that measures the blood to detect dis-ease. |
| Compression Garments<br>BodyMagic<br>www.ardysslife.com/<br>madisoncarlista | BodyMagic garments are the best on the market for compression wear. The garments were designed by one of the world's top orthopedic surgeons and a team of medical engineers. |
| eXfuze Seven | Acai / Gac / |

| | |
|---|---|
| Anti-Oxidant Liquid | Seabuckthorn / Noni / Mangosteen / Gogi / Fucoidan |
| | Benefits: Cleaning and Detox |
| LeVive<br>Anti-Oxidant Liquid<br>www.ardysslife.com/<br>madisoncarlista | Acai / Gogi / Noni / Mangosteen / Pomerganent |
| Life Ionizer<br>Alkaline Water Filter<br>760-585-1608<br>Thai@earthtrade.com<br>www.lifeioniers.com<br>*It is best to call Life Ionizer to place your order. Ask for* **Thai Cabados**. *Very personable!*<br>*Mention S2O and get an additional 10% off of your unit(s).* | Produces Alkaline Water for consumption as well as Acid water for skin and hair care. Acid water is also excellent for cleaning fruits & veggies. |
| UltraStream DIY Colon Hydrotherapy Unit<br>Go to<br>*www.madisoncarlista.com*<br>to get more information and order the unit. | Compact and conveniently portable self administered colon irrigation simple for anyone to use. You can have all the benefits of internal cleansing. Certification is not required to administer the treatment or order the unit. |

| National Vaccine Information Center www.nvic.org | The National Vaccine Information Center (NVIC) is dedicated to the prevention of vaccine injuries and deaths through public education and to defending the informed consent ethic. As an independent clearinghouse for information on diseases and vaccines, NVIC does not promote the use of vaccines and does not advise against the use of vaccines. They support the availability of all preventive health care options, including vaccination, and the right of consumers to make educated, voluntary health care choices. POWERFUL WEBSITE! |
|---|---|

| Natures Squatting Platform for Bowel Elimination<br><br>http://www.naturesplatform.co.uk/index.php | Diseases of the bowel in two thirds of the world's population are rare. The only thing they do differently, from us westerners, is they squat when they answer the call of nature.<br>In India, China and Japan majority of population squat to eliminate. These cultures have a wide range of diet. The problem of diseases of the bowel is to do with what is NOT eliminated. |
| --- | --- |

| Gaia Saunas http://www.gaiainfrared saunas.org/ | These saunas are very therapeutic, relaxing and by far the most beautiful saunas I have ever seen. Gaia saunas, G-Series are elegant and very easy to assemble. The price – AFFORDABLE! |
|---|---|

Be sure to log onto www.madisoncarlista.com for more information and referrals. As I grow and come into more information, I will share it with you.

# Meet the Author

Nine years ago, Madison Carlista was given a diagnosis of advanced cervical cancer with a prognosis of 3-6 months. Without surgery, drugs, chemotherapy or radiation, 8 years later she is whole, healthier and more vibrant than ever.

Madison came to understand the body's amazing ability to cure and heal itself, provided it is facilitated with a balanced environment including but not limited to an organic whole food diet, clean water and internal cleansing and a lot of self love and appreciation. Since overcoming her challenge, she still employs many of these same practices as a lifestyle regimen to support her anti-aging.

Madison is a colon hydrotherapist, naturopathic wellness coach, dynamic edutainment speaker and now inspirational author. Before coming into the alternative wellness industry, she was a marketing communications specialist holding various high profile positions with major sports, entertainment and Wall Street financial firms, such as the NBA, EMI, and Zurich Scudder Investments. Her accomplishments span across the country and she is renowned for her personal and professional network connections and unique Zen-like approach to business.

Her mission in life is to play and have fun. Madison has started and played a major role in several successful entrepreneurial endeavors. She has co-creating non-profit organizations, hosted radio talk shows and positioned her influence in the business development of holistic wellness spas and a fitness facility.

She has just launched two live interactive internet television shows, $S^2O$ and Between the Sheets that airs on www.s2oAgency.com. Madison is also working on the development of $S^2O$ Spa Institute for Anti-Aging and Holistic Healing, a new approach to beauty and wellness.

Madison is an avid workout enthusiast, book collector, professed social network junkie and perpetual student of life, business and world leadership with strong admirations for T. Harv Eker, Paul Zane Pilzer and Blair Singer.

Madison now lives in Atlanta, Georgia. As a single mother she raised her adult daughter to be a beautiful and forward thinking young woman and an inspiration and role model to other youth.

The best way to truly experience Madison's story and her passion is to have her personally speak to your group or organization. You will expand on the insight in this book by learning:

- How to permanently change your aging blueprint for natural and lasting wellness.
- A detailed step by step process for reversing sickness, dis-ease and aging so that you are truly living in the lifestyle.
- Rarely revealed secrets that the medical community is not willing to openly share.
- The underlying cause of obesity and weight gain.

- How to release your hidden emotional blocks that can speed your body's immune system.
- How to recognize your "wellness personality" so you can build on your strengths and overcome your body's weaknesses.

Madison is available for speaking engagements. If you would like her to share her story with your women's group, faith-based organization or other gathering, you can contact her at www.MadisonSpeaks@madisoncarlista.com.